PREOPERATIVE AND POSTOPERATIVE DERMATOLOGIC SURGICAL CARE

PREOPERATIVE AND POSTOPERATIVE DERMATOLOGIC SURGICAL CARE

Hubert Thornton Greenway, Jr., M.D.
Head, Mohs Micrographic Surgery and Cutaneous Oncology
Division of Dermatology and Cutaneous Surgery
Scripps Clinic and Research Foundation
La Jolla, California

Terry Lee Barrett, M.D.
Director, Dermatopathology Fellowship Program
Naval Medical Center, San Diego and
Scripps Clinic and Research Foundation
La Jolla, California

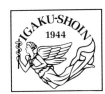

Igaku-Shoin   New York • Tokyo

Published and distributed by

IGAKU-SHOIN Medical Publishers, Inc.
One Madison Avenue, New York, New York l0010

IGAKU-SHOIN Ltd.,
5–24–3 Hongo, Bunkyo-ku, Tokyo 113–91.

Library of Congress Cataloging-in-Publication Data

Preoperative and postoperative dermatologic surgical care / [edited
    by] Hubert Thornton Greenway, Jr., Terry Lee Barrett.
        p.   cm.
    Includes bibliographical references and index.
    ISBN 4-260-14261-5
    1. Skin—Surgery.   2. Preoperative care.   3. Postoperative care.
4. Postoperative Care.   I. Greenway, Hubert T.   II. Barrett, Terry
Lee.
    [DNLM: 1. Skin Diseases—surgery.   2. Ambulatory Surgery—methods.
3. Preoperative Care.   WR 140 P927 1995]
RD520.P74   1995
617.4′77—dc20
DNLM/DLC
for Library of Congress   94-22504
                                                           CIP

ISBN: 0-89640-261-4   (New York)
ISBN: 4-260-14261-5   (Tokyo)

Printed and bound in the U.S.A.
10   9   8   7   6   5   4   3   2   1

PREFACE

The practice of dermatologic surgery is both a science and an art requiring education, training, proficiency and experience. Both the scope and complexity of cutaneous surgical procedures have increased as we seek to provide the best of care for our patients.

This text has been planned to assist the office based cutaneous surgeon. While basic surgical skills can be learned in training sessions such as cadaver laboratories and in real life situations at the operating table, to achieve the most successful outcome also requires specific preoperative planning and meticulous postoperative care.

Preoperatively the surgeon must consider many factors including the appropriate evaluation and informed consent. The necessary equipment must be available which in the vast majority of cases, means an in office procedure and operating arena. The exact nature of the procedure must be planned in advance which includes a knowledge of the anatomy and a plan for anesthesia, primarily local anesthesia.

When tissue is removed for pathologic examination and interpretation, the surgeon must be able to understand pathology techniques and the limitations of those techniques. The surgeon must be able to communicate appropriately the results of this examination. Preoperative planning includes a determination of what type of procedure is most likely to yield an optimal specimen for histologic examination.

Postoperative care will often separate an acceptable from an excellent final result. Wound and postoperative care must be specific and coordinated with the patient. Complications do occur and must be recognized and dealt with appropriately.

Dermatologic surgery requires a team approach and the nursing staff must and do contribute not only intra-operatively but also during the preoperative evaluation and postoperative care periods. The relationships extablished between the patient and nursing staff are critical to a successful outcome.

Procedural skills can be learned with practice and training. Judgement requires experience which of itself empties the hour glass. We hope that with thoughtful preoperative planning and appropriate postoperative care the cutaneous surgeon can provide the best in dermatologic surgery and it is to that effort that this work has been assembled.

Hubert T. Greenway, Jr. M.D.

Terry L. Barrett, M.D.

FOREWORD

Preoperative and Postoperative Dermatologic Surgical Care has been designed as a practical guide for the practicing dermatologist. Drs. Greenway and Barrett have selected an outstanding group of contributors, many of whom are involved in active clinical practice and research. They include not only physicians but nurses, clinic coordinators and attorneys, all equally important in a satisfactory patient outcome.

As patients become more intimately involved with the understanding and participation of their care, the importance of the preoperative evaluation and postoperative care cannot be overemphasized. In fact, these are the two areas where the patient most actively participates for a given surgical procedure.

The text begins with the necessities of an appropriate preoperative evaluation and the informed consent, the latter increasingly important as physicians have a duty to adequately disclose details so that patients can make intelligent and rational decisions regarding their care.

The importance of presurgical and postsurgical nursing care, postoperative care as wound healing occurs months after suture removal, and complications from surgery are also discussed in depth, the latter often dependent on the patient perception of the final result.

The book is directed mainly toward the practicing dermatologist, but other physicians involved in cutaneous surgery including head and neck surgeons, plastic surgeons, ocular surgeons, general surgeons, and family physicians, will find this book of great value. Practical aspects are stressed throughout and many suggestions for patient care, instructions that may be used to increase patient involvement and satisfaction with a procedure are included.

Dr. Greenway has had extensive experience in all areas covered by the text by virtue of his position as Head of Mohs Surgery, Division of Dermatology and Cutaneous Surgery, Scripps Clinic and Research Foundation, and the multiple boards and task forces that he serves on in matters relating to dermatologic surgery. He is board certified in Dermatology, Family Practice, and Mohs Micrographic Surgery.

Dr. Barrett, a dermatologist, pathologist, and dermatopathologist is the Director of the Naval Medical Center-Scripps Clinic and Research Foundation Dermatopathology Fellowship Program. He has a special interest in helping the physician match the planned surgery with the pathology of the tumor to obtain the best results for the patient.

Drs. Greenway and Barrett are the authors of multiple publications and innumerable presentations to medical students, dermatology residents, fellows, and practicing physicians in preoperative and postoperative surgical care for the dermatologic patient.

Roger Cornell, M.D.
Senior Consultant in Dermatology
Scripps Clinic and Research Foundation
La Jolla, California

ACKNOWLEDGMENTS

The many gracious contributors who provided their practical knowledge and experience have made this publication a reality. To them many thanks are expressed.

Special mention is due to two of our teachers whose stimulation encouraged our efforts. Frederic E. Mohs, M.D. has set the standard in the field of cutaneous neoplasm surgery. James H. Graham, M.D. with his experience and vast knowledge of both the pathologic and biologic nature of skin tumors encourages us to seek the best of surgical care for the maximum benefit of our patients.

Sincere appreciation is extended to Deanna Himelright for typing and organizing much of the manuscript.

Our wives, Colleen and Trish, have been most gracious in their support and kindness and to them we are most thankful.

Hubert T. Greenway, Jr. M.D.

Terry L. Barrett, M.D.

CONTRIBUTORS

Terry Lee Barrett, MD
Director, Dermatopathology Fellowship Program
Naval Medical Center, San Diego and
Scripps Clinic and Research Foundation
La Jolla, California

J. Greg Brady, DO
Mohs Surgeon
Allentown, Pennsylvania

Eric A. Breisch, PhD
Department of Pathology
Children's Hospital
San Diego, California

Robert A. Cosgrove, Esq.
Attorney-at-Law
Consultant, Scripps Clinic and
    Research Foundation
La Jolla, California

Ira C. Davis, MD
Instructor of Dermatology
Wake Forest University Medical Center
Department of Dermatology
Winston-Salem, North Carolina

Hubert Thornton Greenway, Jr, MD
Head, Mohs Micrographic Surgery and Cutaneous
    Oncology
Division of Dermatology and Cutaneous Surgery
Scripps Clinic and Research Foundation
La Jolla, California

Christine M. Hayes, MD
Associate Professor
Department of Dermatology
University of Iowa
Iowa City, Iowa

Dudley Clarke Hill, MB, FACD
Dermatologic and Mohs' Surgery
Adelaide, Australia

David E. Kent, MD
Clinical Instructor
Department of Dermatology
Medical College of Georgia
Augusta, Georgia

Barry Leshin, MD
Associate Professor of Dermatology
    and Otolaryngology
Wake Forest University Medical Center
Department of Dermatology
Winston-Salem, North Carolina

D J Papadopoulos, MD
Co-Head, Mohs Surgical Division
Department of Dermatology
Emory University Medical School
Atlanta, Georgia

Judith A. Plis, BS, MBA
Clinic Coordinator
Mohs' Surgery and Cutaneous Laser Unit
Scripps Clinic and Research Foundation
La Jolla, California

Nancy L. Vargo, RN
Oregon Health Sciences University
Department of Dermatology
Portland, Oregon

Duane C. Whitaker, MD
Professor and Director of Dermatologic Surgery
Department of Dermatology
University of Iowa
Iowa City, Iowa

Marilynn J. Winters, RN M.S.
Attorney-at-Law
San Diego, California

Avis B. Yount, MD
Clinical Instructor
Department of Dermatology
Medical College of Georgia
Augusta, Georgia

CONTENTS

1

PREOPERATIVE EVALUATION

Avis B. Yount, MD

Surgical outcomes depend not only on the technical aspects of the surgery, but on careful planning. Preoperative evaluation has several goals: (1) evaluation of the problem to be treated surgically, (2) patient education about the disease process, (3) explanation of the proposed procedure and alternative treatments, (4) risks that may occur because of the procedure, (5) evaluation of underlying medical problems that may lead to complications, (6) basis for obtaining informed consent, (7) discussion of preoperative preparation, postoperative care and limitations, and (8) reduction in patient anxiety.[1,2]

Preoperative assessment benefits both the patient and the physician. The patient becomes involved, and there is a better understanding of the procedure. This builds a good foundation for informed consent. By assessing the potential complications and reducing patient anxiety, the procedure is less stressful for both the patient and the physician.

Surgical procedures in dermatology are most often performed for cutaneous neoplasms, but other procedures include dermabrasion, chemical peels, laser surgery, liposuction, hair transplantation, and nail surgery. If the problem to be treated surgically is a cutaneous malignancy, then the type of tumor and its location, size, and histology need to be evaluated for adequate surgical planning.[2] The patient needs to be educated concerning the disease process, the actual procedure, postoperative care, and limitations. It is important to determine whether preoperative sedation or sedation anesthesia in addition to local anesthesia is needed. This will determine if someone needs to accompany the patient to the procedure and what type of care may be needed postoperatively. The advantages of one type of treatment versus other treatment alternatives should be discussed. The risks of the procedure (e.g., infection, bleeding, and possible nerve damage) should be explained. The patient needs to understand that a scar will result from the procedure[3] and that occasionally a second procedure is needed to improve the contour of the scar.

A good history and physical examination are the best measures for screening for underlying medical problems in patients undergoing surgery. The history and clinical findings, not the laboratory testing, most often change the operative plans.[1] Underlying cardiac problems, particularly in the elderly, can be assessed as well as the need for antibiotic prophylaxis, discontinuance of anticoagulants, and wound healing problems.

Questionnaires such as in Figure 1-1 can be very useful. A history of underlying diseases such as hypertension, cardiac disease, diabetes, liver disease, and renal disease can be obtained.[2,4,5] A review of systems can elicit wound healing problems and bleeding abnormalities.[2,4] Knowledge of the patient's previous history of hospitalizations, surgeries, hepatitis, blood transfusions, and radiation is helpful. Also important is knowledge of the presence of glaucoma, artificial lens, artificial joints, use of contact lenses, and history of other dermatologic disorders such as psoriasis, atopic eczema, and herpes simplex.[3]

Allergies to drugs such as antibiotics, narcotics, and antiseptics and what type of reaction should be documented. A history of current medications, including both prescription and nonprescription drugs such as aspirin and nonsteroidal anti-inflammatory agents, is helpful in determining potential bleeding problems and drug interactions. It is important to review the smoking history, especially when a graft or flap is anticipated, and alcohol intake history for determining potential bleeding problems and drug toxicities. Also, the patient's occupation or job description as it relates to physical activity and sun exposure may need to be considered for postoperative planning.

The physical examination for most dermatological procedures is limited to the problem to be treated. Blood pressure, pulse, and respiration determinations may be important for screening for hypertension, arrhythmias, and lung disease. Documentation of the size and location of tumors, neurological defects in the area, and lymphadenopathy is needed. Simple visual acuity testing should be done for procedures involving the eye. Examination of scars and other dermatologic disorders such as herpes simplex infection and bacterial infection is helpful. Examination of skin tension lines and the laxity of the skin is useful in planning possible flaps, grafts, and closures of defects. Photodocumentation can be obtained at this time.

Laboratory studies depend on whether the patient has any underlying abnormalities that need to be evaluated, such as arrhythmias or bleeding tendencies. CAT or MRI scans may be needed to determine lymph node involvement or involvement of underlying bone. Testing for hepatitis B and HIV may be appropriate for procedures such as dermabrasion. The anesthesiologist may request certain tests for the patient undergoing sedation or general anesthesia. Usually this testing includes hemoglobin, hematocrit, BUN, glucose, serum potassium, and, if the patient is over the age of 40, EKG.[1]

Name: Date:

Telephone: (   )

Age: Height: Weight:

In order that we may better understand your entire health picture, we ask that you fill out this form about the state of your health at this present time.

State of Health: Excellent   Good   Fair   Poor
(Circle)

Drug Allergies:

Are you currently taking any of the following medications?

                                        Yes   No   Date Last Taken

Coumadin
Insulin
Antibiotics
Digoxin
Steroids
Aspirin

Please list all other medications or drugs, including over-the-counter drugs, you are taking at the present time.

Medications and Dosage:

Do you have or have you ever had any of the following conditions?

                                                                Yes   No

Diabetes
Heart Trouble
          Heart Surgery
          Irregular Heartbeat
          Rheumatic Fever
          Pacemaker
          Artificial Heart Valve
Asthma or Lung Problems
Bleeding Tendency
Blood Clots
Hepatitis or Liver Problems
Glaucoma
Arthritis
High Blood Pressure
Kidney Trouble
Cancer
Seizures or Epilepsy
Atopic Eczema
Artificial Joints
Blood Transfusions

Do you smoke?   Yes _____ No _____
          How Many Years? _____   Packs per day _____

Do you drink alcoholic beverages:
          Yes _____   No _____   Drinks per day _____

Previous Hospitalizations:

Previous Surgical Procedures:

Previous Skin Cancers:

Have you ever had any excessive bleeding following minor cuts or dental procedures?

Have you or any of your family ever had any unusual reactions to general anesthesia as elevated temperature or difficulty in awakening?

Have you ever had any reactions to local anesthetics?

Figure 1.1.   Preoperative health questionnaire

Table 1.1.   ASA Physical Status Classification[6]

I. Healthy—no organic or other abnormalities
II. Mild to moderate systemic disease
III. Severe systemic disturbances
IV. Life-threatening severe systemic disorders
V. Moribund patient

ASSESSMENT OF THE OPERATIVE RISKS

The American Society of Anesthesiologists classifies patients into five categories according to their general medical or physical condition (Table 1-1).[6] Usually Class I and Class II patients can undergo outpatient anesthesia without any problems.[7] Class I consists of healthy individuals without physiological, psychological, or organic disorders. Class II patients have only mild to moderate diseases such as mild diabetes, controlled hypertension, and nonlimiting or slightly limited organic heart disease. Also included in this category are the elderly, neonates, heavy cigarette smokers, and patients with chronic bronchitis.[8] Because many dermatologic procedures use local anesthesia, some Class III patients may be able to undergo certain procedures.[4] Class III patients have underlying disorders such as severe diabetes, cardiovascular complications, severe pulmonary insufficiency, and severely limiting organic heart disease.

UNDERLYING CARDIAC ABNORMALITIES

Goldman and his coworkers studied cardiac risk factors in patients undergoing noncardiac surgery with general anesthesia. The two most significant factors were uncompensated congestive heart failure and a history of myocardial infarction within the last six months. Other factors included age over 70, aortic stenosis, and an abnormal cardiac rhythm, especially in patients with more than five premature ventricular contractions per minute. Smoking, hypertension, stable exertional angina, mitral valve disease, cardiomegaly, and conduction system disease did not correlate with increased cardiac risk.[9] However, patients with conduction system disease can be at increased risk because of the underlying cardiac disease.[8] Also, in noncoronary surgery, the operative risk for the patient with a history of coronary bypass surgery at least one month prior to the operation is the same as for patients without coronary artery disease.[10] Even though these cardiac risks have been studied mainly in patients undergoing general anesthesia, they can be used as guidelines to evaluate the severity of underlying cardiac disease in patients undergoing outpatient surgery.

A systolic blood pressure of more than 150 mm Hg and a diastolic pressure greater than 100 mm Hg are associated with more frequent hematoma formation.[11] Elliot and Stein studied the effects of local anesthesia with epinephrine in 40 patients with atherosclerotic heart disease undergoing oral surgery and could not find any significant changes in blood pressure, heart rate, and the electrocardiogram.[12] The total dose of epinephrine in an average healthy adult should not exceed .3 to .5 mg or 30 to 50 mL of 1:100,000 solution over a 30-minute period.[13] Diuretics may cause hypokalemia leading to arrhythmias and increased sensitivity to the effects of epinephrine.[2,4]

Idiosyncratic reactions to the combination of epinephrine and propranolol leading to malignant hypertension, bradycardia, and cardiac arrest have been reported.[14] Epinephrine is an α-1, β-1, and β-2 agonist. The β-2 vasodilatory effects predominate over the α-1 vasoconstrictive effects. However, propranolol is a β-1 and β-2 antagonist; theoretically, with the β blockade, the vasoconstrictive effect of epinephrine is unmasked, leading to hypertension and vagal reflex bradycardia.[15] This could potentially cause cardiac arrest or a cerebrovascular accident. However, Dzubow did not find any significant change in blood pressure with the use of both drugs in patients undergoing Mohs surgery.[16] A decrease in the amount of epinephrine, using a different anesthetic and slower injection over a longer period of time, and blood pressure monitoring may be helpful. Also, patients with hepatic or renal dysfunction may be more susceptible to the effects of lidocaine because of decreased metabolism and excretion of the drug.

It must be remembered that patients with cardiac pacemakers have significant underlying cardiac disease. It is possible for electrosurgical devices to interfere with the function of cardiac pacemakers. There are two types of pacemakers: fixed-rate and demand pacemakers. Most patients today have demand-type pacemakers, and the most common type of demand pacemaker is a ventricular inhibited type. Because of this, electromagnetic radiation (as from an electrosurgical unit) may be sensed by the pacemaker and interpreted as a ventricular beat. With prolonged use, this could lead to pacemaker inhibition and subsequently to bradycardia or asystole. Fortunately, most pacemakers have an outer metallic covering that shields the pacemaker from stray electromagnetic radiation as well as internal protective circuitry.[17,18]

When electrosurgical devices are used in patients with pacemakers, it is best to use as low a setting as possible, place the ground as remotely as possible from the pacemaker and the heart, avoid the use of the active electrode near the pacemaker or the heart, and avoid cutting currents except in a setting with cardiac monitoring and resuscitation equipment. It is also recommended that short bursts of current less than five seconds in duration be used with a 10-second rest period.[17,18] Bipolar forceps can be used more safely because there is less distance between the active and inactive electrodes. The pulse and level of consciousness should be monitored throughout the procedure, and some patients may require cardiac monitoring.[9,18] If electrocoagulation is going to be extensive, a magnet can be taped over the pacemaker to convert it to an asynchronous mode to avoid intermittent inhibition. In some patients, the pacemaker may also need to be checked postoperatively to ascertain if it is functioning properly.[19]

Electrosurgery should be avoided in unstable patients with pacemakers. Alternatives to electrosurgical devices for coagulation are thermal cautery, carbon dioxide laser, vessel ligation, and the ultrasonic scalpel. There are also patients who have implanted defibrillators; the use of electrosurgical devices should be avoided in these patients.

EVALUATION OF BLEEDING PROBLEMS

Prolonged bleeding leads to the terrible triad of hematoma formation, infection, and dehiscence. Any personal or family history of prolonged bleeding after minor cuts or dental procedures, or excessive nosebleeds needs to be investigated. A history of drugs used, such as aspirin, nonsteroidal anti-inflammatory agents, warfarin, or vitamin E, and a history of alcohol intake need to be obtained. Not only is alcohol a vasodilator, but patients with alcoholic liver disease may have a prolonged prothrombin time (PT). A complete blood count (CBC), platelet count, prothrombin time, partial thromboplastin time, and bleeding time will give adequate information in most cases.

A prothrombin time obtained the day of surgery that is below 15 to 17 seconds, with a mean normal value around 11 seconds, is probably adequate to prevent excessive bleeding.[20] An elective incisional biopsy can be done in patients with thrombocytopenia if the platelet count is greater than 50000, and a small punch biopsy can be done if the platelet count is greater than 10000.[21] Heparin is used in hemodialysis, and because heparin has a short half-life of four hours, surgery can be done on a day when the patient is not having dialysis.

Aspirin and related drugs are probably the major cause of bleeding problems in dermatologic surgery. Aspirin is mainly used to prevent complications from coronary artery disease and arterial vascular disease, and to treat arthritis. In the majority of patients, except for patients using high-dose aspirin for rheumatoid arthritis, aspirin can be temporarily discontinued. Aspirin inhibits cyclooxygenase, which blocks the pathway to thromboxane A_2. Thromboxane A_2 is necessary for formation of the platelet plug to stop blood loss from capillaries, small arterioles, and venules.[22,23] Even one baby aspirin is sufficient to inhibit platelet function. This inhibition by aspirin is irreversible and remains for the life span of the platelet, which is 7 to 10 days. Aspirin needs to be discontinued 7 to 14 days prior to the surgery and can be restarted one day after the surgery.[22,23]

Nonsteroidal anti-inflammatory agents inhibit thromboxane synthetase; inhibition occurs only when the drug is circulating. Therefore, their action is dependent on the half-life of the drug, and these drugs should be discontinued one to four days prior to the surgery.[22,23]

Dipyridamole (Persantine) is a platelet adhesion inhibitor and a vasodilator. Some feel that this drug does not cause significant bleeding problems, but others feel that it needs to be discontinued two to three days prior to surgery.[4,22,23]

Warfarin (Coumadin) interferes with vitamin K–dependent coagulant proteins II, VII, IX, and X. These proteins are necessary for fibrin formation or secondary hemostasis. These factors are more important in large- vessel hemostasis, particularly bleeding that occurs hours to days after surgery.[22,23] The physician who prescribed the warfarin may need to be consulted before discontinuing the drug. Patients at low risk for discontinuing the warfarin are those treated for deep-vein thrombosis and cerebrovascular accident prevention. Patients at high risk for problems caused by the discontinuance of warfarin are those with hypercoagulable states and those with prosthetic heart valves.[23] In low-risk patients, the warfarin can be stopped three days before surgery and resumed one day after surgery at the regular dose. For high-risk patients, the warfarin can be discontinued one week prior to surgery and the patient given heparin, 5000 units IV, followed by 15000 to 20000 units subcutaneous (SQ), then 8000 to 10000 units SQ every eight hours or 15000 to 20000 units every 12 hours. On the day of surgery, the patient is given 5000 units SQ twice a day. The day after surgery, the full dose of heparin is resumed and the warfarin restarted. The heparin is discontinued when adequate coagulation is obtained with the warfarin.[22] Surgery can be done on the patient given warfarin, but more bleeding will develop if the prothrombin time is twice the mean normal value, the surgery is on the scalp, and the patient is hypertensive.[19] A prothrombin time can be obtained one to two weeks before surgery and the dose of warfarin adjusted to the lowest dose to obtain a therapeutic response.[22]

ANTIBIOTIC PROPHYLAXIS

Prophylactic antibiotics may be used as an adjunct to help prevent wound infection.[22] Risk factors associated with surgical wound infection in dermatologic surgery include prolonged length of the surgery, impaired wound healing as seen in diabetics, the operative site, and active infection at another site. In addition, operative technique and preparation of the site preoperatively can play a role in wound infection.[22,24]

Prolonged length of the procedure in the range of three or more hours, as frequently occurs with Mohs' micrographic surgery, may increase the risk of wound infection.[22] Impaired wound healing can be seen in patients with diabetes mellitus, underlying malignancy, obesity, malnutrition, immunosuppression, and age over 70.[22,24] In diabetics, there is defective chemotaxis and response to bacteria.[2] Blood glucose levels higher than 300 mg/mL are associated with an increased risk of infection.[4] Surgery in certain anatomic sites such as the axillae, perineum, and mouth; active infection at another site distant to the operative site; and surgery on inflamed cysts are also risk factors for infection.[22,24] A noninfected but ulcerated tumor, particularly at such sites as the ear, and reexcision of crusted biopsy sites may increase the chance for infection.

Recommendation for prophylaxis in dermatologic surgery can be made from considering the preceding factors, the type of bacteria likely to cause the infection, and what has been determined from studies in general surgical procedures. The time of prophylactic antibiotic administration and risk for wound infection has been studied in patients undergoing elective general surgical procedures.[25] Administration of parenteral antibiotics two hours before the procedure significantly reduced the wound infection rate. Antibiotics given one to four hours after the surgery did not reduce the risk of infection, and the incidence was the same as for patients not given any antibiotics.[25]

Haas and Grekin,[26] in a review on antibiotic prophylaxis in dermatologic surgery, recommend the use of a single preoperative dose in most cases; for prolonged cases they would consider a postoperative dose six hours after surgery. If there is a significant risk of infection, the antibiotics could be used for 24 hours postoperatively (Table 1-2). Salasche suggested that antibiotics could be started 24 hours prior if given orally or two hours preoperatively if given parenterally[22] and could be continued for one to two days because this will protect against bacterial entry until the epithelial migration covers the

Table 1.2. Recommendation for Antibiotic Prophylaxis in Prevention of Wound Infection[26]

	1 Hr Preop	6 Hrs Postop
Dicloxacillin	1 gm po	500 mg po
1st-generation cephalosporins	1 gm po	500 mg po
Clindamycin (penicillin allergy)	300 gm po	150 gm po

wound.[22] It is probably best to use antibiotics for as short a period as possible, and only in the case in which the wound may already be infected as in an inflamed cyst or a tumor with clinical inflammation would antibiotics be considered the day before surgery. In this incidence, antibiotics are being used to treat infection prior to surgery and not being used for prophylaxis.

Dicloxacillin or a first-generation cephalosporin would be the choice of antibiotics because these cover most staphylococcus aureus infections. For procedures near the external ear canal, prophylaxis with Ciprofloxacin may be preferred because of the possibility of *Pseudomonas aeruginosa* infection in this area.

Antibiotic prophylaxis for bacterial endocarditis is recommended for dental, upper respiratory, gastrointestinal, and genitourinary procedures.[27] However, the need for prophylaxis in dermatologic surgery has not been studied as well. A recent article by Fang et al. on prosthetic valve endocarditis following nosocomial bacteremia found that *Staphylococcus epidermidis* and *Staphylococcus aureus* were the most common cause of endocarditis in patients after bacteremia.[28] The most common portals of entry of the bacteria were intravascular catheters and wound and skin infections. Fine et al. reported significant bacteremia following incision and drainage of abscesses and recommended antibiotic prophylaxis.[29] Sabetta and Zitelli found an 8.4% incidence of bacteremia during surgery for noninfected but ulcerated tumors of the skin. Bacteremia was not observed in skin surgery in tumors with intact skin.[30] Most likely the incidence of bacteremia is low in skin surgery, particularly when done on intact skin.

The American Heart Association recommends endocarditis prophylaxis for patients with prosthetic cardiac valves, rheumatic and other acquired valvular disorders, mitral valve prolapse with valvular regurgitation, most congenital cardiac malformations, and hypertrophic cardiomyopathy.[27] Wagner et al. have recommended antibiotic prophylaxis for these patients undergoing dermatologic procedures such as curettage and incisional and excisional surgery. It is felt that prophylaxis should be directed toward staphylococcal infections with the use of first-generation cephalosporins or Dicloxacillin.[31] Table 1-3 shows suggested recommendations for dermatologic surgery.

Table 1.3.   Endocarditis Prophylaxis in High-Risk Patients for Dermatologic Surgery[31]

Dicloxacillin	2 gm po 1 hour preop	1 gm po 6 hours after initial dose
1st-generation cephalosporin	1 gm po 1 hour preop	500 mg po 6 hours after initial dose
Penicillin allergy Erythromycin stearate	1 gm po 2 hours preop	500 mg po 6 hours after initial dose
or Erythromycin Ethylsuccinate	800 mg po 2 hours preop	400 mg po 6 hours after initial dose

In patients with artificial joint replacement undergoing dental procedures, the use of prophylactic antibiotics has been controversial. Orthopedic surgeons often recommend prophylaxis in patients who have ulcerated infected wounds or an infection of the skin at a distant site. A first-generation cephalosporin is the recommended agent because it is effective not only for gram-positive organisms but for 50% of gram-negative organisms.[20]

WOUND HEALING EVALUATION

Wound healing can be delayed in patients with underlying medical disorders such as uremia, anemia, poorly controlled diabetes mellitus, malignancy, vascular insufficiency, autoimmune disorders, and Ehlers-Danlos.[32] After age 70, there is a decrease in tensile strength in wounds. Delayed healing is also seen in patients on chronic corticosteroids. 40 mg of Prednisone daily is more likely to cause problems with wound healing, whereas 10 mg of prednisone daily will have a minimal effect.[20] Transplant patients may have problems with wound healing because of the use of immunosuppressant drugs. A history of recurrent herpes simplex infection on the lip in an area where surgery is to be performed can delay healing and cause more scarring and therefore the patient should have prophylaxis with acyclovir.

A knowledge of the patient's history of hypertrophic scarring or keloid formation is important. Perioperative intralesional corticosteroids and the use of silastic gel sheeting can be considered. Hypertrophic scars are more common on the chest, and this should be explained to the patient prior to surgery.

Recently several articles have studied the effect of cigarette smoking on flap and graft survival. Cigarette smoking decreases the tissue oxygen level because of vasoconstriction.[33] One study demonstrated that skin flap survival was significantly decreased in nicotine-treated animals except when nicotine was withheld for two weeks before the surgery.[34] Goldminz and Bennett found in a retrospective study that the use of flap and graft necrosis was related to the number of packs of cigarettes smoked per day. Necrosis was less in nonsmokers and those who smoked less than one pack per day. Goldminz and Bennett recommended advising the patient to decrease smoking to less than a pack per day for two days before surgery and at least one week after surgery to help maintain an adequate blood supply to the flap or graft.[35]

CONCLUSION

Preoperative evaluation is beneficial to both the patient and the physician. Through patient evaluation, the patient has a better understanding of the disease process, the surgical procedure, potential risks, and postoperative management. With a good knowledge of the patient's history and a pertinent physical examination, the physician can evaluate the underlying disease process and medical problems and plan the procedure. Potential problems related to current medications, bleeding problems, wound healing problems, underlying diseases such as cardiac disease and hypertension, and the need for antibiotic prophylaxis can be addressed. Education of the patient and management of these potential problems before the surgery help lead to a successful outcome for both the patient and the physician.

REFERENCES

1. Roizen MF, Rupani G. Preoperative assessment of adult outpatients. In: White PF, ed. Outpatient Anesthesia. New York, NY: Churchill Livingstone, 1990:181–200.
2. Leshin B, Whitaker DC, Swanson NA. An approach to patient assessment and preparation in cutaneous oncology. *J Am Acad Dermatol.* 19:1081–1088; 1988.
3. Bennett RG. Fundamentals of Cutaneous Surgery. St Louis, MO: CV Mosby; 1988:357–361.
4. Proper SA, Rose PT. Preoperative evaluation of the Mohs surgery patient. In: Mikhail GR, ed. Mohs Micrographic Surgery. Philadelphia, PA: WB Saunders; 1991:174–183.
5. Elliott DL, Tolbe SW, Milker SH, et al. Medical considerations in ambulatory surgery. *Clin Plast Surg.* 10(2):259–307, 1983.
6. Schneider AJ. Assessment of risk factors and surgical outcomes. *Surg Clin North Am.* 63:1113–1126, 1983.
7. Dripps RD, Eckenhoff JE, Vandam, LD: Introduction to anesthesia: Principles of Safe Practice. 7th ed. Philadelphia, PA: WB Saunders; 1988:15–16.
8. Elliott DL, Linz DH, Kane JA. Medical evaluation before operation. *West J Med.* 137:351–358, 1982.
9. Goldman L, Caldera DL, Nussbaum SR, et al. Multifactorial index of cardiac risk in noncardiac surgical procedures. *N Engl J Med.* 297:845–850, 1977.
10. Crawford EC, Morris GC, Howell JF, et al. Operative risk in patients with previous coronary artery bypass. *Ann Thorac Surg.* 26:215–221, 1978.
11. Courtiss EH, Kanter MA. The prevention and management of medical problems during office surgery. *Plast Reconstr Surg.* 85:127–136, 1990.
12. Elliot GD, Stein E. Oral surgery in patients with atherosclerotic heart disease: Benign effect of epinephrine with local anesthesia. *JAMA.* 227:1403–1404, 1974.
13. Marten TJ. Physician-administered office anesthesia. *Clin Plast Surg.* 18:882, 1991.
14. Foster CA, Aston SI. Propranolol-epinephrine interaction: A potential disaster. *Plast Reconstr Surg.* 72:74–78, 1983.
15. Winton GB. Anesthesia for dermatology surgery. *J Dermatol Surg Oncol.* 14:41–54, 1988.
16. Dzubow LM. The interaction between propranolol and epinephrine observed in patients undergoing Mohs surgery. *J Am Acad Dermat.* 15:71–75, 1986.
17. Bennett RG. *Fundamentals of Cutaneous Surgery.* St Louis, MO: CV Mosby; 1988: 357–361.
18. Sebben JE. Electrosurgery and cardiac pacemakers. *J Am Acad Dermatol.* 9:457–463, 1983.
19. Furman S, Hayes DL, Holmes DC. *A Practice of Cardiac Pacing,* 2d ed. Mount Kisco, NY: Future Publishing Co; 1989: 603–604.
20. Krull EA. Patient evaluation for dermatology surgery. In: Roenigk RK, Roenigk HH, eds. *Dermatologic Surgery Principles and Practice.* New York, NY: Marcel Dekker; 1989:51–61.
21. Robinson JK: *Fundamentals of Skin Biopsy.* Chicago, IL: Year Book of Medical Publishers, 1986.
22. Salasche SJ: Acute surgical complications: Causes, prevention and treatment. *J Am Acad Dermatol.* 15:1163–1185, 1986.
23. Goldsmith SM, Leshin B, Owen J. Management of patients taking anticoagulants and platelet inhibitors prior to dermatologic surgery. *J Dermal Surg Oncol.* 19:578–581, 1993.
24. Lichtor JL. Premedication for adult outpatients. In: White PF. *Outpatient Anesthesia.* New York, NY: Churchill Livingstone; 1990: 201–225.
25. Classen DC, Evans SR, Pestotnik SL, et al. The timing of prophylactic administration of antibiotics and the risk of surgical wound infection. *N Engl J Med.* 326:281–286, 1992.

26. Haas AF, Grekin RC. Antibiotic prophylaxis in dermatologic surgery. Accepted for publication in *J Am Acad Dermatol*, 1994.

27. Dajani AS, Bisno AL, Chung KJ, et al. Prevention of bacterial endocarditis: Recommendations by the American Heart Association. *JAMA*. 264:2912–2922, 1990.

28. Fang G, Keys TF, Gentry LO, et al. Prosthetic valve endocarditis resulting from nosocomial bacteremia. *Ann Intern Med*. 119:560–567, 1993.

29. Fine BC, Sheckman PR, Barlett JG. Incision and drainage of soft tissue abscesses and bacteremia. *Ann Intern Med*. 103:645, 1985.

30. Sabetta JD, Zitelli JA. The incidence of bacteremia during skin surgery. *Arch Dermatol*. 123:213–215, 1987.

31. Wagner RF, Grande DJ, Feingold DS. Antibiotic prophylaxis against bacterial endocarditis in patients undergoing dermatologic surgery. *Arch Dermatol*. 122:799–801, 1986.

32. Bennett RG. *Fundamentals of Cutaneous Surgery*. St Louis, MO: CV Mosby; 1988:80–81.

33. Jensens JA, Goodson WH, Hopf HW, et al. Cigarette smoking decreases tissue oxygen. *Arch Surg*. 126:1131–1134, 1991.

34. Forrest CR, Pang CY, Lindsay WK. Pathogenesis of ischemia necrosis in random-pattern skin flaps induced by long-term low-dose nicotine treatment in the rat. *Plast Reconstr Surg*. 87:518–528, 1991.

35. Goldminz D, Bennett RG. Cigarette smoking and flap and full-thickness graft necrosis. *Arch Dermatol*. 127:1012–1015, 1991.

2

INFORMED CONSENT

Robert A. Cosgrove Esq.

Marilynn J. Winters, RN, MS

INTRODUCTION

The doctrine of informed consent can be one of the more confusing and disquieting legal issues that physicians today face in their daily practice. In the traditional practice of medicine, the physician's opinion was held in such high regard that it was accepted and relied upon without question by the patient.[1] Those times are gone. Today the watchwords are self-determination, consumerism, and informed consent.

Courts and legislatures have imposed a duty on the physician to adequately disclose details regarding contemplated procedures, treatments, or surgeries so that the patient can make an intelligent and rational decision whether to undergo such care. Unfortunately, "adequate disclosure" has not been uniformly defined. Thus, the informed consent process can be confusing.

Moreover, issues related to informed consent may arise even before treatment has begun. Consequently, a claim for medical negligence on the grounds of lack of informed consent may be raised notwithstanding otherwise competent, acceptable medical care.[2]

In the past, dermatologists were at low risk for medical malpractice claims. As the practice of dermatology has expanded to include more surgical procedures (scar revisions, skin grafts, flaps, cancer excisions, and cosmetic procedures) the risk of malpractice claims has increased.[3] Correlatively, the need to understand the requirements and ramifications of "informed consent" becomes imperative. This chapter will address the development of the concept of informed consent, its general legal criteria, impediments to the informed consent process, and risk management issues. This chapter is a general overview only. It is not intended as a definitive statement of the law in any particular state or jurisdiction. For specific advice, please consult with an attorney specializing in medical malpractice defense in your jurisdiction.

HISTORICAL PERSPECTIVE

Early case law focused on whether or not the patient agreed to go forward with the contemplated procedure. In essence, the courts utilized a battery theory of analysis that asked whether consent to touching had occurred. For example, in *Mohr v Williams*[4] the patient consented to a left ear surgery. The physician, while in surgery, found the pathology greater in the right ear and performed surgery on that ear instead. Although the surgery was medically sound, the patient sued and prevailed.

In the seminal case, *Schloendorff v Society of New York Hospital*,[5] Justice Cardozo, an eminent and respected jurist, set forth what has become the cornerstone of the doctrine of consent:

> Every human being of adult years and sound mind has a right to determine what shall be done with his own body. . . .[6]

In *Schloendorff*, the patient consented to an examination under anesthesia. During the examination, the physician found a tumor and removed it. Following the removal of the tumor, the patient suffered complications that required amputation of her fingers. The patient sued for battery and was successful.

As case law evolved, it became apparent that the battery theory of analysis would not adequately cover more complex and involved circumstances. This was particularly true as the courts' focus became whether consent was informed.

In 1957, a California court of appeal introduced the phrase "informed consent." In *Salgo v Stanford University*,[7] the patient suffered a paralysis after a thoracic aortography. The patient alleged that he was not told of the risks. The court, in finding for the patient, held that uninformed consent was not true consent and that "[a] physician violates his duty to his patient . . . if he withholds any facts which are necessary to form the basis of an intelligent consent by the patient to the proposed treatment."[8] The court also recognized that disclosure of all risks was sometimes unwise and that some discretion on the part of the physician was appropriate.[9] Thus, the court did not define the parameters of an "adequate disclosure."

Three years later, the Kansas Supreme Court, in *Natanson v Kline*,[10] attempted to set forth guidelines for adequate disclosure. The patient in that case had received severe radiation burns and skin breakdown following radiation therapy after a mastectomy for cancer. The court held that the physician was obligated to make a reasonable disclosure to the patient concerning the nature and probable consequences of the proposed treatment as well as the dangers that the physician knew were incident to or possible in the treatment rendered. The court also required that the physician discuss with the patient the nature of the ailment, the nature of proposed treatment, the probability of success, and alternatives.

By 1972, the California Supreme Court abandoned the battery approach in lieu of a negligence theory of analysis. The court held that if a physician fails to meet his duty to disclose pertinent "material" information, the action is based in negligence.[11] The court also required that known risks of death or serious bodily harm be disclosed as well as information the patient considered material to the decision.

CURRENT STATE OF THE LAW

Under traditional law the physician merely explained the nature of the procedure and then obtained the patient's consent to proceed.[12] Such an approach is no longer legally acceptable. Today, informed consent is a process consisting of dialogue between patient and physician where information is exchanged, questions are asked, and answers are given. An informed decision on if and how to proceed is then made by the patient.

Each participant has certain responsibilities. The patient must provide accurate historical information and complete details regarding current complaints. The patient must also question when information given is unclear. Reciprocally, the physician must learn what is important to the patient in order to properly tailor disclosure of risks and benefits.

The development of the process of informed consent is based on at least three factors: (1) the patient's growing awareness of his or her right to know, (2) the avalanche of cost containment procedures, and (3) the public's recognition that physicians are fallible.

ELEMENTS OF INFORMED CONSENT

The parameters of adequate disclosure and the standard by which the disclosure of information is judged varies from state to state. Most jurisdictions, however, agree that the following general areas should be covered with the patient: diagnosis, nature and purpose of the procedure or treatment, expected outcome and probability of success, material risks, benefits and consequences, alternatives and their supporting information, and the effect that nontreatment has on prognosis and outcome.[13]

Although most courts require the preceding information to be given without asking, a few jurisdictions require less. Before 1987, Georgia, pursuant to statutory law, required that a physician need only explain the intended result of the procedure unless the patient asked for additional information. In 1987, the Georgia legislature expanded the duty of informed consent in certain limited procedures (any surgical procedure involving general, spinal, or major regional anesthesia, amniocentesis, and x-rays requiring intravenous or intraductal contrast media). For such procedures, the physician must disclose material risks as defined by statute.[14] In Oregon, the physician is required to explain the procedure and the existence of risks and alternatives in very general terms. The physician is then duty bound to ask the patient if additional information is necessary. If so, then further disclosure occurs.[15]

Hawaii and Texas have established administrative agencies to standardize the information that must be given before medical or surgical procedures.[16]

DISCLOSURE REQUIREMENTS

Jurisdictions vary on how much information is required for adequate disclosure. Indeed, it is in this area that most litigation occurs.[17]

Overall, states follow one of two standards by which the physician's disclosure is measured: the "professional standard" and the "patient- oriented" standard. The professional standard was first enunciated in *Natanson v Kline*.[18] This standard is based on the premise that the physician, with a high degree of training and experience in complex matters, is in a superior position to know what is best for the patient. Thus, the physician is required to impart sufficient information to the patient as other physicians would in the same or similar community to allow the patient to make an intelligent and rational decision.[19] Expert testimony establishing this standard is required.[20]

Under this standard, the issue before the court is whether the physician's judgment comported with accepted community professional practice. The patient's needs or opinions are not considered. Difficulties arise when there is no consensus as to what risks and options should be discussed. By way of example, a nationwide survey of 100 dermatologists was conducted regarding what treatment options should be discussed with patients concerning four different diagnoses. That survey revealed that the disclosure practices varied widely and "perhaps inappropriately."[21]

By the 1970s, many courts and legislatures began to recognize that the professional standard was inconsistent with the patient's right to make health care decisions. A District of Columbia circuit court was the first to articulate a patient-oriented standard of disclosure.[22] The court embraced the concept that a person has the right to determine his or her own course of medical treatment, and must be afforded an informed choice. Recognizing that the patient's knowledge of medicine was less than a physician's, the court noted the patient could only turn to the physician for advice. In order to uphold the right of self-determination, the court concluded that the standard should not come from the physician. The California Supreme Court in *Cobb v Grant*,[23] adopted this minority standard of disclosure as well. The trend toward adoption of the patient-oriented standard has continued.

The patient-oriented standard requires the physician to disclose information that would be considered significant or material in the decision-making process. It does not require full disclosure of all possible risks and alternatives, but does require adequate or reasonable disclosure so that a patient can make an intelligent and rational decision. For example, with the diagnosis of recurrent basal cell carcinoma, treatment options may include Mohs' micrographic surgery, wide excision, and/or radiation therapy. The advantages and disadvantages of each treatment modality could be determinative for the patient. Thus, each treatment modality would be evaluated based on anticipated functional and cosmetic impairment as well as outcome.[24]

The patient-oriented standard is measured by the patient's need to know. The role of the expert witness in litigation is therefore different than under the professional standard approach. Expert testimony is used to prove the existence of risks, their likelihood of occurrence, and the resulting harm. "Unless the risk is serious and expert testimony can establish its existence, nature and likelihood of occurrence, the risk is not material . . ." and therefore no requirement of disclosure exists.[25] Once the materiality of the risk is established, however, it is up to the jury to decide whether the disclosure should have been made.[26]

In making a determination as to whether the risk is material, the jury uses an objective criterion. A risk is material when a reasonable person would be likely to attach significance to the risk in deciding whether to forego the proposed therapy.[27] A minority position uses a subjective criterion to determine whether the risk is material. Under this approach the patient's individual circumstances are taken into account in determining whether a risk would be construed by that patient as material.

The subjective approach has been condemned on several grounds. First, it requires the physician to inform each individual patient of all possible risks that could influence the patient's decision. In effect, the physician must anticipate an individual patient's idiosyncracies and internal beliefs. This approach also allows the disgruntled patient to testify with 20/20 hindsight, in an often self-serving manner, as to what would have been material. Lastly, it is unsatisfactory to resolve the issue of materiality based on patient credibility alone.[28]

PLAINTIFF'S BURDEN OF PROOF

In order to recover on a theory of lack of informed consent the plaintiff[29] must prove: (1) the physician had a duty to disclose certain risk information and failed to do so; (2) the plaintiff suffered injury from the undisclosed risks; (3) the plaintiff would have refused the procedure or surgery had the risk been properly disclosed; and (4) the plaintiff was injured because of the physician's lack of disclosure.[30]

The causation issue is decided on either an objective or subjective standard, depending on the jurisdiction. Under the objective standard, which most courts use, the analysis is again based on the reasonable person standard. As one court aptly stated:

> If disclosure of all material risks would not have changed the decision of a reasonable person in the position of the patient, there is no causal connection between non-disclosure and his damages. If, however, disclosure of all material risks would have caused a reasonable person in the position of the patient to refuse the surgery or therapy, a causal connection is shown.[31]

A minority of jurisdictions utilize the subjective standard, which takes into account the plaintiff's own judgments and justifications for going forward with the procedure.

EXCEPTIONS TO INFORMED CONSENT

As a general rule, there is no duty to disclose information that is common knowledge. Nor is there a need to disclose information to a patient who already knows such information. Furthermore, one need not disclose information that is irrelevant to the decision making process.[32] Additionally, three general exceptions to disclosure exist: emergency, waiver, and therapeutic privilege.

Emergency

When a physician is confronted with a patient who is incapacitated and unable to give consent, in a life-threatening position requiring immediate intervention, disclosure is unnecessary as to the treatment rendered. In other words, there is insufficient time to obtain consent, and the harm from the failure to treat is imminent and outweighs the harm threatened by the procedure.[33] The basis for this exception is the presumption that a reasonable person would have consented.[34]

Waiver

Waiver occurs when the patient voluntarily, and under no influence, knowingly gives up his or her right to be informed about the benefits, risks, and alternatives to a procedure or surgery before it is done. It is felt that the concept of waiver does not conflict with a patient's right of self-determination. For example, in some instances the patient may realize an inability to deal with the stress involved in treatment discussions and choose not to be subjected to it. By waiving such discussion, preferably in writing, the patient remains in control. The physician's duty under these circumstances is to make sure the patient understands the right to be fully informed.[35]

Therapeutic Privilege

Therapeutic privilege allows a physician to make less than full disclosure when the information would have a deleterious effect upon the patient's emotional condition.[36] Thus, where the information given would cause a person to be so ill or emotionally distraught so as "to foreclose a rational decision, or complicate or hinder the treatment, or perhaps even pose psychological damage to the patient," the physician can keep the information from the patient.[37] Because such action goes against a patient's right of self-determination and ability to make informed decisions, the privilege should be used in very limited circumstances. Otherwise it would engulf and swallow the doctrine.[38] The physician who asserts the therapeutic privilege should document in the patient's chart the emotional state at the time, a summary of the medical findings to justify the use of the privilege, the content not divulged, the rationale for not disclosing, and what was disclosed.[39]

IMPEDIMENTS TO INFORMED CONSENT

Patients who are well informed, as a rule, do better in the postoperative/posttreatment period. Anxiety is decreased, progress occurs at a faster rate, and management of their care is smoother. They are more compliant with instructions, cope better with complications, and express greater satisfaction with results.[40]

Fully informing patients, however, is not always an easy task. Patients may misunderstand or distort what they hear, passively defer to physician judgment, or fail to remember what they were told in the preprocedure/presurgical discussions.

A survey conducted for the President's Commission for the Study of Ethical Problems in Medicine and Biomedical and Behavioral Research revealed that 94% of the respondents wanted to be told everything, both positive and negative.[41] In spite of the need to know everything, when observed, patients who had been given information and treated as the decision-maker more often than not acted in a passive manner, allowing the physician to make the decision.[42]

Most of the patients we interviewed and observed talking with staff of the hospital seemed to want information primarily to know what to expect next and otherwise seemed content to let doctors make decisions. . . . In our observations, we found about 10 (out of 200) patients, depending on how one draws the line, who were very interested in actively involving themselves in decision-making.[43]

Many studies done to test retention of information given preoperatively raise doubts about the patient's ability to recall the information once the procedure or surgery is done. One study of 20 patients undergoing cardiac procedures revealed that when retention of preoperative information was tested four to six months after the procedure, primary recall was 29% and secondary recall (after suggestion) was only 42%. The poorest scores were in the category of potential complications (primary recall was 10% and secondary recall was 23%).[44]

Another study of 100 preoperative and emergency-room patients revealed an overall retention level for information given preoperatively of 35%. These patients had been told that they were part of a study and would receive important information specific to them. They would then be asked about the information at a later date. The study concluded that even with deliberate attempts to obtain informed consent, there is no assurance that a patient can retain the pertinent information given for even one week, despite the patient's claims to understand it at the time.[45]

In a study of 20 facelift patients, all patients remembered being told of the possibility of complications. On further questioning only three patients could remember as many as three potential complications, eight patients could remember only one potential complication and nine patients were either unwilling or unable to recall any specifics.[46] In explaining the lack of recall, one half of the women denied that such a complication could happen to them, or they admitted purposefully putting such complications out of their minds. Others explained their lack of recall by identifying their conviction that they were insulated from such complications. Only two of the patients mentioned that the possibility of complications frightened them, thus explaining their lack of recall.[47]

Another factor that may influence what a patient hears and understands is the patient's motive for the procedure or surgery. One such study revealed that if the decision to have the procedure was based on social, traditional, or religious reasons, the medical information was ignored. Indeed, in this study parents were given detailed information related to their newborn babies' circumcision. Those who selected the procedure based on traditional or religious reasons became angry with their physician for providing detailed medical information concerning the procedure. The impact of this study reinforces the need for the physician to know patient motives and expectations. It also supports the waiver exception to disclosure in that some patients deal with adverse complications by not dealing with them at all.[48]

RISK MANAGEMENT MEASURES

Patient Physician Rapport

The physician must establish and maintain good patient relations. This is critical, as litigation often arises out of circumstances where injury occurs coupled with a breakdown in communications. Examples of faulty communication include (1) physician unavailability, (2) physician/staff unresponsiveness to inquiries, (3) poor bedside manner, (4) a perception that the physician is not truly listening, and (5) disagreements surrounding billing issues and practices.

The Process of Informed Consent

In carrying out the process of informed consent, a verbal discussion should occur between the patient and the physician responsible for the surgery. The procedure, alternatives, risks, and benefits should be discussed in clear and understandable language. As an adjunct to the verbal discussion, a written checklist may be used to assist in the process. The patient should be given a copy of the checklist, with the original placed in the medical chart.

Other techniques can be used to enhance recall, (ie, handouts, pamphlets, videotapes, and tests or verbal questioning to validate the patient's understanding). The consent form can be sent home with the patient to review prior to signing with instructions to write down any questions that may exist.

If photographs are used, they should show a variety of outcomes so that a claim cannot be made that the photographs created unrealistic expectations. Such photographs would reinforce the fact that complications can and do occur.[49] If any adjuncts or visual aids are used, documentation should be maintained to identify the date of usage so that retrieval, if necessary, is possible.

The medical chart should reflect the substantive areas discussed. Overzealous medical documentation can create an inference that a certain risk or alternative not listed was not discussed. Thus it has been suggested that the better practice is to document the general categories that were discussed as part of the informed consent process.

There is no simple solution or one correct method to obtain informed consent. Each practitioner must develop a process that works, taking into account his or her own communication style. Whatever style of communication is adopted, a well-documented medical chart goes a long way in protecting the physician against an allegation of lack of informed consent.

CONCLUSION

The concept of informed consent is an evolving process. It mandates active participation by both the patient and the physician. The goal is to achieve a well-informed, well-reasoned decision by the patient.

REFERENCES

1. Comment. The doctor knows best? Patient capacity for health care decision making. *Oregon Law Rev.* 71:909–937, 1992.
2. Shugrue R, Linstromberg K. The practitioner's guide to informed consent. *Creighton Law Rev.* 24:881–928, 1991.
3. Redden E, Baker D. Coping with the complexities of informed consent in dermatologic

surgery. *Dermatol Surg Oncol.* 10:111–116, 1984. *See also* Altman. survey of malpractice claims in dermatology. *Arch Dermatol.* 111:641–644, 1975.

4. 95 Minn 261, 104 NW 12 (1905).
5. 211 NY 125, 105 NE 92 (1914).
6. 211 NY at 129–130, 105 NE at 93.
7. 154 Cal.App.2d 560, 317 P.2d 170 (1957).
8. 154 Cal.App.2d at 578; 317 P2d at 181.
9. Id.
10. 186 Kan 393, 350 P2d 1093 (1960).
11. *Cobbs v Grant*, 8 Cal.3d 229, 502 P.2d 1 (1972).
12. Wecht C., ed. *Legal Med Annu.* 1985:147.
13. Duffy D, Romney M. Medicine and law: Recent developments in peer review and informed consent. *Tort & Insurance Law J.* 26:331–352, 1991; Shugrue, supra note 2 at 922.
14. *Robinson v Parrish*, 720 F2d 1548 (CA 11 Ga. 1983); Ga Code Ann § 88-2906, 88-2906.1 (1990).
15. Wecht C, ed. (previously mentioned) note 12 at 149 (1985); Ore Rev Stat Ann Title 52 § 677.097 (1992).
16. Hw Rev Stat Chpt 671 § 671-3 (1985); Tex Rev Civ Stat Ann 4590i § 6.03, 6.04 (Vernon Supp 1993).
17. Wecht C, ed. note 12, at 148.
18. 186 Kan 393, 350 P2d 1093 (1960).
19. Studer M. The doctrine of informed consent: Protecting the patient's right to make informed health care decisions. *Montana Law Rev.* 48:85–100, 1987; Merz J, Fischhoff B. Informed consent does not mean rational consent. *J Legal Med.* 11:321–350, 1990.
20. Shugrue (previously mentioned), note 2, at 900, 901.
21. Shriner D, Wagner R Jr, Weedn V. Informed consent and risk management in dermatology: To what extent do dermatologists disclose alternate diagnostic and treatment options to their patients? *J Contemp Health Law Policy* 8:137–162, 1992. (The four diagnoses surveyed were dysplastic nevus syndrome, recurrent basal cell carcinoma, malignant melanoma, and neonatal port-wine stain.)
22. *Canterbury v Spence*, 464 F2d 772 (DC Cir) *cert denied* 409 U.S. 1064 (1972).
23. *Cobb v Grant*, 8 Cal.3d 299, 502 P2d 1.
24. Shriner (previously mentioned), note 21, at 149.
25. Duffy (previously mentioned), note 13 at 349.
26. *Brown v Dahl*, 41 Wash. App. 565, 705 P.2d 781 (1985); Studer, supra, note 19, at 94.
27. *Canterbury v Spence*, 464 F.2d 772, 785 (DC Cir 1972).
28. Wallach D, Berry S. Informed consent in Texas: A proposal for reasonableness and predictability. *St Mary's Law J.* 18:835–882, 1987.
29. Plaintiff is the party who files the professional negligence action. Under a lack of conformed consent theory, typically the plaintiff is the patient.
30. Duffy D (previously mentioned), note 13, at 347.
31. *Sard v Hardy*, 281 Md 423, 450, 379 A2d 1014, 1025 (1977).
32. *Canterbury v Spence*, 464 F2d 722, 788 (DC Cir 1972).
33. Wecht C, ed. (previously mentioned) note 12 at 151.
34. Kukafka A. Informed consent in law and medicine: Autonomy v paternalism. *NY State Bar J.* 61:48–57, 1989.
35. Shugrue (previously mentioned), note 2 at 908.
36. Shugrue at 905.
37. *Canterbury v Spence*, 464 F2d 772, 789 (DC Cir) *cert denied*, 409 US 1064 (1972).
38. Id.
39. Rozovsky F. *Consent to Treatment a Practical Guide.* 2nd ed. Little Brown and Company; 1990:86, 87.

40. Redden E (previously mentioned), note 3, at 112.
41. Redden E, Baker V, Mersel A. The Patient, the plastic surgeon, and informed consent: New insights into old problems *Plast Reconstr Surg.* 75:270–276, 1985. See also Baker J, Kolin I, Bartlett E. Psychosexual dynamics of patients undergoing mammary augmentation. *Plast Reconstr Surg.* 53:652–659, 1974.
42. Redden (previously mentioned), note 48, at 272.
43. Redden, quoting from Lidz C, Meisel A. Informed consent and the structure of medical care. In: the President's Commission for the study of ethical problems in medicine and biomedical and behavioral research . . . 2:317–399, 1982.
44. Robinson G, Merav A. Informed consent: Recall by patients tested post-operatively. *Ann Thoracic Surg.* 22:209–212, 1976.
45. Leeb D, Bowers D Jr, Lynch J. Observations on the myth of "informed consent." *Plast Reconstr Surg.* 58:280–282, 1976.
46. Redden (1984), supra, note 3, at 113; Goin M, Bdurgoyne R, Goin J. Face-lift operation: The patient's secret motivations and reactions to informed consent. *Plast Reconstr Surg.* 58:273–279, 1976.
47. Goin (previously mentioned), note 46 at 277–278.
48. Christensen-Szalanski J, Boyce W, Harrell H. Circumcision and informed consent—is more information always better? *Med Care.* 25:856–867, 1987.
49. Greenberg G. Lipoplasty: The informed consent and medicolegal considerations. *Clin Plast Surg.* 16:375–379, 1989. Hoffman S. Reduction mammoplasty: A medicolegal hazard? *Anesth Plast Surg.* 11:113–116, 1987.

3

SURGICAL FACILITY AND EQUIPMENT

Ira C. Davis, MD

Barry Leshin, MD

INTRODUCTION

The surgical facility and equipment are the foundation of the dermatologist's surgical practice. The dermatology resident begins training in an established facility. The thought dedicated to physical plant design and surgical equipment selection have been determined. Upon completion of training, the trainee is confronted with establishing his own facility and buying equipment. This chapter introduces the practitioner to considerations in the design of the facility and selection of equipment necessary to perform basic dermatologic surgery.

SURGICAL FACILITY

A specific area in the office suite must be dedicated to dermatologic surgery. Although this room may serve as an examination room, an examination room is inadequate for dermatologic surgery. Planning considerations include special needs for electricity, plumbing, lighting, communication, and storage. Designated clean and dirty utility areas to accommodate the surgery unit are essential. Finally, the interrelationship of this space to the nonsurgical patient care areas requires forethought to maximize the patient's comfort and the physician's efficiency.

The Planning Stage

A well-designed surgical area requires considerable planning. Tobin recommends reviewing many existing plans as well as visiting other offices.[1] Personal observations and discussions with physicians and their staff should help delineate the strengths and weaknesses of various designs. The handbook of the Accreditation Association of Ambulatory Health Care, Inc. (AAAHC) identifies standards for accreditation of ambulatory surgery facilities and can be a valuable guide in the designing process.

Patient Care Area

The area devoted to surgery should be the largest subarea among the spaces devoted to patient care. The minimum recommended size ranges from 140 to 200 square feet, with 280 square feet considered ideal.[1,2,3] The resulting size of rooms may necessarily be smaller due to unexpected circumstances such as structural support, plumbing, air-conditioning, and other needs. The number of surgical rooms required relates to the type and volume of procedures anticipated. Cost considerations may limit the full equipping of each surgery room. In such instances, shared equipment should be selected based on its movability. The doorway should be wide enough so that a stretcher can pass through in the event of an emergency. Furthermore, an evacuation route from the surgical space to the outside of the building that will accommodate a stretcher should also be considered. Attention to basic construction materials is essential. A vinyl wall covering or certain washable painted surfaces are desirable to facilitate cleaning walls. For similar reasons, vinyl floor covering should be specified rather than carpeting.

Utilities

Electricity, plumbing, and communications systems may require special consideration in the planning of the surgical suite. Emergency power receptacles or a generator for equipment and lighting need to be planned in case of power failure. In addition, anticipation of location of equipment and electrical outlets will help prevent later problems with current overload. A wall-mounted kick plate in the room allows the surgeon to call for assistance while gloved. Our system consists of a beep and a flashing light over the door to alert other office staff to our needs. We avoid telephones or intercoms in the surgery suite to avoid startling the patient or the physician.

Millwork

The millwork functions as the preparation, storage, and handwashing area for the surgical facility. Factors to consider include countertop height and surface material, sink location, and the relationship of the millwork to the surgical table (Figure 3-1). Our rooms have the millwork behind the recumbent patient. This allows for easy access to the cabinet and countertop from either side of the table. Furthermore, it permits activity that may heighten patient anxiety, such as filling up a syringe, to be out of the patient's view. Glass panels in the upper cabinets permit easy visualization of equipment and supplies for rapid access.

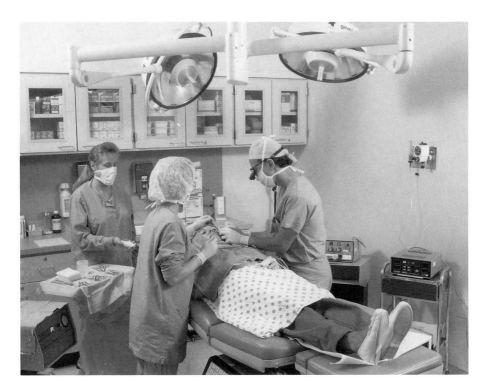

Figure 3.1.   The surgical suite. Note the location of the millwork in relation to the patient.

Surgical Lights

Lighting must adequately illuminate the surgical field and provide an evenly lit
and homogeneous pattern. Patient comfort is a paramount consideration, and the delivery of cool light aids in this process. Furthermore, heat from overhead lights may
increase intraoperative bleeding.

Factors to consider when selecting surgical lights include light intensity, heat production, glare, color correction, field size, and maneuverability.[3] The bulb and filters
will determine the intensity of the light. The heat produced is a function of bulb type,
filter, and venting. In addition, the larger the dish size the less heat emitted. Reflective
lighting reduces shadow and glare. Filters aid in maintaining an accurate tissue color,
which is helpful for photodocumentation. Field size correlates directly with the dish
diameter. Dish concavity determines focal distance of the light from the patient.

The delivery system should be easily reachable, movable, flexible, and stable.
Sterilizable or disposable handles are an option for the surgeon if intraoperative light
manipulation is important. Ceiling-mounted lights are the best option. Track lighting
offers the greatest maneuverability. Other options include wall-mounted or freestanding lights. Freestanding lights allow for mobility; however, they utilize precious floor
space. Wall-mounted lights are not as easily maneuverable.

Operating Tables and Stools

The paramount factor in operating-table selection is patient and surgeon comfort. The physician should lie on the table before purchase. In addition, the table should be power operated and allow for separate lift, back, foot, and tilt maneuvers. Programmable tables permit pushbutton and time-saving access to predesignated positions. Chairs, in contrast to tables, allow for easier access to the head and neck areas. Armboards and stirrups are essential features.

Some surgeons may prefer performing procedures while sitting. Hand or foot air-lift or manually adjustable stools with and without back support are available. The air-lift stools are significantly more expensive but can be easily adjusted while the physician is gloved.

Suction

The importance of suction in the control of vigorous bleeding cannot be overstated. Suction may be attached to the wall with the collection device in a separate area from the operating-room suite. More commonly, a portable suction device such as the Gomco unit is adequate for the dermatologic surgeon.

Waste Disposal

Removal of contaminated waste is an integral component of safety in the work environment. Kick-bucket waste containers or plastic-lined plastic receptacles should be placed in a convenient location. The waste should be packaged in biohazard bags and disposed of in accordance with OSHA regulations regarding safe disposal of contaminated waste.

Occupational Safety and Health Regulations

OSHA regulations pertaining to the surgical facility consist of the Hazard Communication regulations and the Bloodborne Pathogens standard. The Hazard Communication regulation was issued in August 1987, followed in December 1991, by the Bloodborne Pathogen standard. The American Academy of Dermatology has distributed excellent manuals to assist its members in compliance with both sets of regulations.[4,5]

The Hazard Communication regulations require employers to evaluate the hazards of all chemicals in the workplace. This information must be transmitted to employees through a Hazard Communication Plan. This document catalogs all hazardous chemicals and contains a compendium of material safety data sheets on the chemicals. Additionally, the plan documents employee training, employee safety, and appropriate labeling of all hazardous chemicals. Chemicals specifically related to a surgical practice would include formalin, chemical peel solutions, hydrogen peroxide, benzoin, ferric subsulfate (Monsel's solution), and Betadine.

The Bloodborne Pathogens standard was developed to protect workers from occupational exposure to blood and other potentially infectious materials. This set of regulations requires the employer to identify which duties may lead to exposure to blood or other potentially infectious materials, and focuses on eight areas: universal precautions, engineering and work practice controls, personal protective equipment, housekeeping, laundry, hepatitis B vaccination and postexposure evaluation and follow-up, communication of hazards to employees, and record-keeping.

SURGICAL ANTISEPTICS

The purpose of prepping the surgical site is to remove pathogenic organisms and to reduce the resident flora to its lowest level. Because 10% to 20% of the resident flora cannot be removed by surgical scrubbing, the skin cannot be completely sterilized. Iodophors and chlorhexidine are the two agents routinely used for preparation of the surgical site.[6] Iodophors are iodine-polymer complexes, of which povidone-iodine (Betadine) is the most common agent. Iodophors' antiseptic property relates to the release of free iodine, which occurs after two minutes of contact time.[7] Betadine Surgical Scrub contains an added detergent. Hibiclens contains 4% chlorhexidine gluconate and 4% alcohol in a sudsing base. Both iodophors and chlorhexidine are effective against a broad range of gram-positive and gram-negative bacteria. In addition, chlorhexidine is effective against various molds, yeasts, and viruses. In the manner typically used in cutaneous surgery, neither agent is effective against spores.

Most comparison studies indicate that chlorhexidine is the most effective antiseptic agent. Chlorhexidine's onset of antiseptic activity is more rapid than the iodophors and is less irritating to the skin. Caution must be used with chlorhexidine near the ear because its passage to the middle ear through a perforated tympanic membrane can result in ototoxicity. Chlorhexidine's sudsing base can also cause conjunctival irritation.

Dzubow and colleagues have demonstrated that a 10-second wipe with 70% isopropyl alcohol in prepackaged pledgets is sufficient in reducing aerobes and anaerobes for procedures lasting less than five minutes on facial skin.[8] They recommend a 10-second alcohol wipe followed by either chlorhexidine or povidone-iodine. A painting of the operative site with povidone-iodine in an alcohol solution for less than one minute is as effective as a five-minute scrub with povidone-iodine detergent followed by a povidone-iodine solution.[9] Takegami and colleagues advocate a clean technique method consisting of a two-second wipe with 70% isopropyl alcohol pad and injection of local anesthetic, followed by a 10-second skin prep with a prepackaged povidone-iodine swab in a circular motion over a minimum area of 6 × 6 cm.[10]

Hair should be removed only when necessary.[7] Clipping (rather than shaving) with electric clippers or the use of a depilatory are the methods of choice. Hair removal should be done just before surgery.

SURGICAL INSTRUMENTS

General Considerations

Excisional surgical instruments are of primary importance to the cutaneous surgeon. The anatomic location of surgeries may determine the specific instrument required. Although initially expensive, high-quality instruments have a longer life. Tungsten carbide inserts in scissors and needle holders permit more precise cutting and needle-holding security, respectively.

Scalpel Handles

Scalpel handles can be divided into two types: the Bard-Parker and Beaver systems. The #3 Bard Parker metal scalpel handle is the type most commonly used in dermatologic surgery. The #4 handle is similar in shape to the #3, but slightly larger, and accommodates a larger blade. The Beaver scalpel handles are more delicate instruments and use smaller scalpel blades. Siegel has designed a scalpel handle that integrates a Beaver-type handle that holds the Bard-Parker scalpel blades.[11]

Scalpel Blades

The scalpel handle selected dictates the blade type. Bard-Parker handles accept Bard-Parker scalpel blades. Similarly, Beaver blades are used with the Beaver scalpel handles. Both carbon steel and stainless steel blades are available, but the former are sharper.

The most common Bard-Parker scalpel blade is the #15. The #15C is a similarly shaped, narrower blade with a more acute taper and can be used for more delicate or smaller excisions.[12] The shape can vary to some degree depending on the manufacturer. The #11 blade is useful for incision and drainage procedures. The #10 blade is a larger blade with a longer cutting surface that is useful in our practice for larger excisions through a thick dermis, such as the trunk. Robinson recommends the #10 blade for shave removal of larger nevi.[13] A #20 or #22 blade, both of which are larger versions of the #10 blade, can also be used on thicker skin.[14] These two blade types, however, require a #4 scalpel handle.

The Personna Plus steel surgical blades have a Teflon microcoating that allows for decreased tissue resistance and drag. They are available in all sizes except for the #15C. However, this manufacturer's #15 blade is somewhat narrower than the standard #15 blade.

The Beaver blades are smaller than the Bard-Parker blades. The #67 is the diminutive of a #15 Bard-Parker blade.

Razor Blades

Razor blades are commonly used for shave biopsies and excisions. The Gillette Super Blue Blade is a carbon steel blade coated with an anticorrosive oil.[15] Sterilization of the blade does not significantly affect its sharpness. The blade may be broken in half in its longitudinal plane. This maneuver, usually done with a blade-breaking instrument, increases the blade's flexibility but decreases its stability. The Personna razor blade, a stainless steel blade, is also effective.

Scissors

General Considerations

Scissors serve a variety of functions in cutaneous surgery. Consequently, different scissors serve specific roles, such as undermining, suture removal, and dressing changes. The scissor can be divided into its component parts: handle, blades, and tips. Handles can vary in length. Longer handles are able to reach longer distances. Shorter handles are useful for more delicate procedures. Blades can be curved or straight.

Curved blades provide better visualization and access for finer work.[16] Scissor tips may be blunt or sharp or have one tip of each type. Blunt tipped blades provide for less traumatic undermining while sharp tipped blades are superior for fine dissection. Blades may be either smooth or serrated. The serration decreases tissue slippage and is useful in thin-skinned areas such as the eyelid.[16] Some scissors are available with angled blades, which are useful in areas of poor visibility such as the external auditory canal or for special procedures. LaGrange scissors are useful for harvesting punch grafts during hair transplantation.

Tissue Cutting-undermining Scissors

Undermining scissors are used for blunt tissue dissection as well as for cutting (Table 3-1). The iris scissor is the prototypical scissor for fine-tissue dissection and cutting. The Stevens tenotomy and gradle scissors have narrower tips than the iris scissor and are preferred by many dermatologic surgeons. Metzenbaum, strabismus, and Mayo scissors have longer handles and wider blades than the more delicate scissors previously mentioned. These features permit more efficient undermining of large or fibrous areas.[3] The Metzenbaum and strabismus scissors can be used for trunk and facial cutaneous surgery. Selection of an iris-Stevens-gradle–type or Metzenbaum-strabismus–type scissor will afford the cutaneous surgeon the ability to undermine and cut tissue for most routine excisional surgical procedures.

Suture Scissors

Specifically designed scissors are available for cutting sutures (Table 3-1). These instruments have a small hook on one of the blades to slip under the suture loop.

TABLE 3.1.   Scissors

Function	Type	Comments
Fine tissue cutting/ undermining	Iris	prototype scissor
	Gradle	more delicate tips, sturdier blades than iris
	Stevens tenotomy	longer blades than gradle, more versatile
Trunk and facial tissue cutting/undermining	Metzenbaum	most useful for large trunk excisions
	Strabismus	smaller and more delicate than Metzenbaum
	Mayo	rarely used in cutaneous surgery
Suture cutting	Northbent	useful for cutting fine sutures
	Shortbent	
	Spencer	
	Littauer	used for 4-0 and larger sutures
	Iris,	alternative to suture scissors
	Gradle	
Bandage cutting	Lister	dressing removal
	Universal	cuts metal, greater cutting power

Data from References #3, 14, 16

Alternatively, iris or gradle scissors can be used for suture removal. Scissors dedicated to tissue undermining and cutting should not be used for cutting sutures because this will decrease the sharpness of the instruments and affect their precision.

Bandage Scissors

Bandage scissors are used for the removal of dressings (Table 3-1). The Lister bandage, Universal bandage, and cloth scissors consist of two angled blades. One blade has a wide blunt tip that can be placed under the dressing without damaging the underlying skin.

Forceps

Forceps are used to grasp tissue. Forceps may be smooth, serrated, or toothed. Most surgeons prefer toothed forceps to grasp tissue because a small amount of tissue can be securely grasped while minimizing crushing of the tissue. Some forceps are available with a suture platform, which aids in grasping the suture needle during closure. Adson and Brown-Adson forceps are the most versatile.[14] For more delicate tissue an iris forceps or a variant of the iris forceps is preferred (Table 3-2). Forceps are avail-

TABLE 3.2.   Forceps

Type	Application
Adson	most versatile forceps
	1 × 2 teeth used for tissue handling
Brown-Adson	similar to Adson
	7 × 7 tooth pattern allows for better control of tissue
Iris	more delicate than Adson
	used for handling thin and delicate tissue
Semken	variants of the iris forceps handle or tips
Stevens	vary from the iris
Bishop-Harmon	
Foerster	
Graefe-Iris	
Paufique	
Jeweller's forceps	fine tips useful for pinpoint electrocoagulation and grasping suture fragments
Carmalt splinter	grasp suture and small pieces of tissue and
Walter splinter	foreign bodies
Graefe-Tissue	grasp cartilage
Dejardin	
Lerner	combination skin hook and forceps differ in
Frankel-Adson	placement of skin hook on forceps
Hudson	

Data from References #3, 14, 16, 17, 18

Table 3.3. Skin Hooks

Type	Application
Cottle	J-shaped tenaculum, single or double hook
Frazier	hook similar to shepard's crook
Tyrell's	smaller version of Frazier
Guthrie	double skin hooks
Joseph	
Stevens tenotomy	blunt tip prevents perforation of delicate tissue

Data from References #14, 16

able for specific situations such as pinpoint electrocoagulation and grasping cartilage or suture. Combined skin hook and forceps are available as well.[17,18]

Skin Hooks

Skin hooks facilitate atraumatic tissue handling. With the recent concern for transmission of infectious disease such as the human immunodeficiency virus, some surgeons avoid skin hooks. There are multiple variations in the shape of the hook and handle as well as the number of prongs. Double-pronged hooks, in contrast to the single-pronged hooks, allow for better visualization of the depth of the wound as well as increased tissue stability.[3,19] The tenaculum tip may be sharp or blunt. Rakes are skin hooks with more than two prongs. Features of specific skin hooks are detailed in Table 3-3.

Needle Holders

Needle holders are composed of the jaw and handle; there are multiple variations in these two components (Table 3-4). Smooth and fine-toothed jaws are available. The smooth jaw is preferable because it does not result in damage to the suture. The size of the suture needle will dictate the type of needle holder used. Tungsten carbide inserts permit better grasp of the needle and a decrease in instrument wear, but their value is questioned by some surgeons.

Hemostats

Hemostats are used to clamp severed vessels before suture ligation or pinpoint electrocoagulation. The hemostat can also be used to remove scalpel blades as well. Hemostats are available with curved or straight tips. The curved-tip hemostats are useful for ligating vessels; their prototype in dermatologic surgery is the Halstead mosquito hemostat (5 in). The Kelley hemostat is longer (5 1/2 in) and is traditionally used in general surgery. This larger instrument has straight tips and is useful for grasping the nail plate while performing nail avulsion.

Table 3.4.   Needle Holders

Type	Features
Webster (4 1/2 to 5 in)	most commonly used for delicate cutaneous surgery
Derf	shorter jaws than Webster
Halsey	longer jaws than Webster
Crile-Wood	longer jaws and handles
Neuro-smooth	Neuro-smooth for smaller needles
Baumgartner	useful for handling needles on #2-0
Mayo-Hegar	and #3-0 suture
Castroviejo	delicate, spring-locked, useful for periorbital surgery
Olsen-Hegar	combination needle holder and scissor
Gillies	

Data from References #14, 16, 20

Punches

Disposable punches are sharp, sterilely packaged, and inexpensive; they have largely replaced reusable punches. Hair transplant punches are available in increments of 0.25 mm and are useful for precise removal of small lesions; they are intermediate in size between the standard disposable punch sizes.[14]

Curettes

Curettes vary in the size and shape of the handle and configuration of the head. Curettes range in size from 1 to 8 mm in diameter. The Fox curette has a slender, square-shaped handle that resembles a pencil. The Piffard curette has a heavy handle and comes in only three sizes (small, medium, large). Smaller curettes such as the Buck, Heath, and Meyerhofer are useful for curetting smaller pockets of tumors or cysts. The Skeele curette has a cup-shaped head with serrations, which is useful for curetting out cyst walls.

Miscellaneous Instruments

Towel clamps can be used to clamp together sterile towels to stabilize the draping of the surgical field. The cord of the electrosurgery handle can be woven through the handle rings and permits easy access of that handle to the surgeon. The Jones and Backhaus towel clamps are commonly used. Allis forceps have a broad clamp surface and are useful for tissue retraction. The Desmarres chalazion clamps can be used on the eyelids and lips to provide a bloodless surgical field as well as tissue stabilization. Periosteal (Freer) elevators or dental spatulas are useful in separating the nail plate from the nail bed and periungual attachments during nail avulsion. An English anvil nail splitter is useful for partial nail avulsions. The Schamberg comedo extractor is most convenient because it is easy to use and clean. Other comedo extractors have lancets on one end. The Zimmerman-Walton has one end in which a disposable hypodermic needle can be placed.

Mayo Stands

Mayo stands allow for placement of instruments or materials in a convenient, accessible manner. Freestanding models with two or four casters are available. A Mini-Mayo wall-mounted unit is available for conservation of floor space.

CARE OF SURGICAL INSTRUMENTS

Introduction

Proper sterilization techniques are essential in the preparation of instruments for dermatologic surgery. The care of instruments can be divided into cleaning, packaging, sterilization, and setup of the surgical tray.

Instrument Cleaning

All foreign and organic debris must be removed from the instrument after each use. This is to ensure that no organisms will be protected during the sterilization process and to prevent any accumulation of debris that might interfere with its future use.[21] Instrument cleansing consists of soaking, scrubbing, rinsing, and lubrication.

The instruments should be soaked in water with a neutral pH detergent immediately after use. Manual scrubbing with a plastic brush can be done. However, ultrasonic cleaners rely on fine bubbles to dislodge debris. These cleaners mitigate employee injury and save valuable time.[22] Visual inspection of the instruments may detect persistence of residual debris that would require brushing and an additional cycle in the ultrasonic cleaner. After cleaning, the instruments are rinsed to remove all the detergent and lubricated with instrument milk or dried thoroughly. Some physicians prefer to use instrument milk only when lubrication is necessary. For more severe instrument stiffness, an overnight soak in 50% ammonia water and 50% isopropyl alcohol solution is useful.

Instrument Packing

The preferred method of instrument sterilization is in packs rather than as loose instruments. Self-sealing or taped paper-transparent packs are the preferred method for office sterilization. The paper-transparent packs remain sterile for up to one year. Although woven and nonwoven cloth packs were thought to remain sterile for only a period of weeks, a recent study indicated that no significant difference was noted when compared to polypropylene peel pouches over the course of 50 weeks.[23] The self-sealing packs are quicker to use and easier to handle.[21] Gauze placed inside the package with the instruments helps to absorb excess moisture. Lockable instruments should be packaged in their unlocked positions. Sharp edges of instruments should not touch each other when autoclaved. Autoclavable protectors are available for instrument tips or for the whole instrument.

Packages should be dated at the time of sterilization and should have indicators to reflect that they have been sterilized.

Instrument Sterilization

Forms of heat sterilization are the primary means of sterilization in the dermatologic surgery practice. This form of sterilization is the most reliable means of destruction of bacteria, viruses, and the more resistant bacterial spores.[22]

The steam autoclave is the most popular means of sterilization in the office setting. It is a reliable and simple method requiring only electricity and distilled water. Metal, paper, cloth, glass, and heat-resistant plastics can be sterilized. The cycle time will vary with the size of the pack, temperature level, and chamber pressure. The average cycle is 45 min.[22] Although the humidity may dull or damage some instruments, this is not a practical concern if high-quality stainless steel instruments are used.[21,22] The width of the device will determine the size of the surgical pack that can be accommodated.[2]

The Chemiclave is a steam autoclave that replaces distilled water with a chemical solution composed of methylketone, acetone, formaldehyde, and three alcohols.

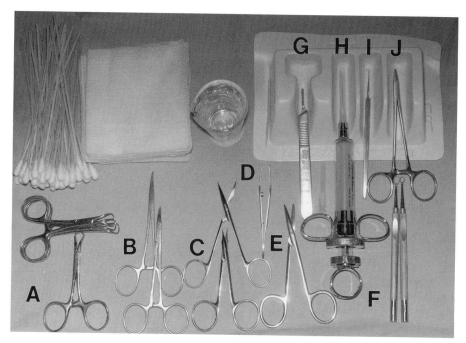

Figure 3.2.   The surgical tray. Sterile cotton-tipped applicators, gauze, shot glass, and toothpick are located at the top left-hand corner of the tray. The shot glass is used as a receptacle for gentian violet. The toothpick is used as a marking pen. Instruments are arranged on the tray as follows: A. Backhaus towel clamps; B. Halstead mosquito curved hemostats; C. curved iris scissor (top), gradle scissor (bottom); D. Paufique forceps; E. Strabismus scissors; F. Rein currettes; G. Bard-Parker #3 scalpel handle; H. 3-ringed, glass 10-cc syringe; I. Frazier skin hook; and J. Webster needle holder. Instruments G-J are in a Preven-A-Stick holder.

Because of the lower humidity the instruments are dry at the end of the cycle and there is less susceptibility to instrument damage due to moisture. Potentially toxic chemical vapors may be released with this device.

Dry-heat sterilization requires more exposure time for sterilization. Cloth, paper, and plastic materials cannot be sterilized. Because instruments cannot be packaged, proper handling of the instruments is problematic. Because there is no moisture, instruments will not be dulled. A small heat sterilizer requiring only 6 min for sterilization of unpackaged instruments may be useful in offices that have small inventories of instruments or a low volume of procedures.[24]

Gas sterilization uses ethylene oxide. This method provides no heat or moisture; therefore, it is an ideal method for heat- or moisture-sensitive instruments. Owing to the toxicity of the gas and length of the cycle, an environment guaranteeing complete aeration is necessary. This method, therefore, is best suited for hospital use.

Cold (chemical) sterilization is not a sufficient method for sterilization of instruments. Glutaraldehyde preparations such as Cidex, Glutarex, Acu-sol, and Sporicidin are the most reliable. These open solutions can become grossly contaminated. They require 7 to 10 hours for destruction of spores.[22] Because the instruments must be rinsed with water after sterilization, this results in the possibility of recontamination.

Surgical Tray Setup

The surgical pack consists of the basic instruments needed for excisional surgery procedures (Figure 3-2). This includes, but is not limited to, a scalpel handle, suture- and tissue-cutting scissors, tissue forceps, skin hook, hemostats, and towel clamps. Instruments not commonly used should be sterilized separately and added to the pack as necessary. In addition, packs for suture removal, punch biopsies, and other common procedures can be designed. A barrier drape should be applied over the Mayo table to allow for a sterile field to place instruments. Ring forceps within the pack are helpful in arranging the other instruments on the tray.[21,22]

WOUND CLOSURE MATERIALS

Sutures

Introduction

No suture exists that can be used for every clinical situation. Therefore, the physician must be familiar with various properties of sutures and choose the best suture for a given situation. Physical and handling characteristics and tissue reaction properties are properties regularly used to choose the appropriate suture.[25,26]

Physical properties of sutures are defined by the *United States Pharmacopeia*. These properties include the suture's physical configuration, tensile strength, caliber, elasticity, plasticity, memory, knot strength, capillarity, and fluid-absorption capability (Table 3-5).

Handling properties of sutures are determined by the material's pliability and coefficient of friction. The coefficient of friction determines tissue drag, degree of knot-tying difficulty, and ease of knot slippage.

Table 3.5. Suture Physical Properties

Property	Definition
Physical configuration	Single (monofilament) or double (multifilamentous) braided or twisted if multifilamentous
Tensile strength	Amount of weight required to break suture increases as suture diameter increases function of specific material
Caliber	Suture diameter Increasing number of zeros (eg, 6-0) results in decreasing caliber
Elasticity	Ability of suture to return to previous configuration after stretching
Plasticity	Ability to remain in its stretched configuration
Memory	Ability to return to its original shape after tying
Knot strength	Force needed for knot to slip
Capillarity	Properties related to the suture when wet
Fluid absorption capability	Determines bacterial colonization of suture

Data from References #25, 26

Tissue reaction properties relate to the host's response to needle injury and the suture material itself. The inflammatory reaction can lead to delayed wound healing, infection, and wound dehiscence.[27] Therefore, the use of the minimal amount and least reactive suture material is critical in preventing complications.

The major suture manufacturers are Ethicon and Davis & Geck. Other manufacturers include Look and S Jackson. These latter two companies provide a shorter biopsy suture measuring 8–10 in, which is cheaper than the conventionally sized 18-in suture.

Absorbable Sutures

Introduction

Sutures are considered absorbable if they lose most of their tensile strength within 60 days. The absorbable sutures most commonly used are polyglycolic acid (Dexon–Davis & Geck), polyglactin 910 (Vicryl-Ethicon), polydioxanone (PDS–Davis & Geck), and polytrimethylene carbonate (Maxon–Davis & Geck). Fast-absorbing gut (Ethicon) is a heat-treated, nonchromic salt containing suture that dissolves rapidly.[28] This suture is used epicutaneously, and is useful for wounds on the face. Its rapid dissolution makes suture removal unnecessary and accounts for its utility in children's surgery, and in securing skin grafts.

Polyglycolic acid (Dexon)/Polyglactin 910 (Vicryl)

These two sutures were the first two synthetic sutures manufactured. Both are braided sutures with similar properties. Coated forms of Dexon marketed as Dexon Plus and Dexon II were introduced for easier handling. The original Dexon has been renamed Dexon S. These sutures are available in dyed and undyed forms.

Polydioxanone (PDS)

This suture differs from Dexon and Vicryl in two important respects. First, it is a monofilamentous suture; therefore, it is less likely to be colonized with bacteria. It also retains its tensile strength longer. It is completely absorbed in 180 days in contrast to 60–90 days and 120 days for Vicryl and Dexon, respectively.[29] This suture is more difficult to handle than the coated Vicryl and Dexons. Polydioxanone II is easier to handle than the original PDS.

Polytrimethylene carbonate (Maxon)

Maxon, a monofilament suture, has a tensile strength similar to that of PDS.[30] However, it is easier to handle. Like PDS, it is more expensive than Dexon or Vicryl. A comparison study of 584 repairs of surgical defects showed no difference in scar width between wounds closed with Maxon or Vicryl.[31] However, Maxon was found to be easier to handle, and no instance of suture breakage was reported. The longer retention of strength of Maxon and PDS may be advantageous when wounds are closed under significant tension.

Nonabsorbable Sutures

Introduction

Nonabsorbable sutures have been traditionally defined as sutures that are not degraded. Strictly speaking, however, some nonabsorbable sutures will eventually be completely degraded. Nonabsorbable sutures commonly used are silk, nylon, polypropylene, braided polyesters, and polybutester.

Silk

Silk is derived from a protein produced by the silkworm larva. This braided suture is soft and easy to handle. It has one of the lowest tensile strengths of any suture and elicits a pronounced inflammatory reaction.[26] Because of its softness, it is useful on mucous membranes and intertriginous surfaces. It is also used to retract tissue and anchor bolsters for grafts because it is unlikely to cheesewire through tissue.

Nylon (Ethilon-Ethicon, Dermalon–Davis & Geck, Surgamid-Look)

Nylon in its monofilamentous form is the most commonly used nonabsorbable suture in cutaneous surgery. Nylon has a high tensile strength and memory, but poor handling and knot security when compared to polypropylene and silk. Three or four knot throws are required to hold each stitch.[26] Nylon tends to cut tissue. The suture is available in green, black, and clear. The green thread aids in visualization of the suture in hair-bearing areas.[25]

Polypropylene (Prolene-Ethicon, Surgilene–Davis & Geck)

Polypropylene has good tensile strength. This suture has a very low coefficient of friction, which makes it ideal for use as a running intradermal stitch. Its knot security is poor and its memory is high, requiring extra throws to retain the knot. Because of its plasticity, the suture stretches during tissue swelling, resulting in less of a likelihood of cutting through tissue. The suture is more expensive than nylon.

Polyesters (Ethibond-Ethicon, Mersilene-Ethicon, Dacron–Davis & Geck)

Polyester sutures such as silks are braided and soft, but have a very high tensile strength. Mersilene and Dacron are uncoated while Ethibond is coated, which decreases tissue drag and triggers less inflammation than the others.[25] This suture's softness accounts for its utility on mucous membrane and intertriginous areas.

Polybutester (Novafil–Davis & Geck)

Polybutester is a monofilament suture designed to have a higher tensile strength, easier handling, and a lower coefficient of friction than nylon or polypropylene.[26]

Suture Needles

Needle selection can be the most confusing aspect of suture selection. The needle itself is divided into three parts: the eye (shank), the body, and the point. The eye is the site of attachment of the suture and determines the size of the suture tract. The body of the needle has a circular shape in cutaneous surgery: 3/8, 1/2, and 5/8 circle needles are available.[2] The most frequently used is the 3/8 circle. The 1/2 or 5/8 circle needles are useful for deep wounds or tight curves. The point is the needle's sharpest portion.

Reverse cutting and conventional cutting needles are used in dermatologic surgery

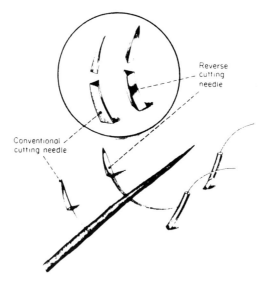

Figure 3.3   Comparison of conventional and reverse cutting needles (with permission from Bennett RG. Selection of wound closure materials. *J Am Acad Dermatol.* 18:632,1988.)

(Figure 3-3). Both needles have triangular tips. Conventional cutting needles have the cutting edges directly laterally and on the inside curve of the needle. Because one cutting edge faces the wound, there may be a higher likelihood of cutting through the tissue with this needle.[25] The PC needle is a conventional cutting needle. The reverse cutting needle has three cutting edges, all directed laterally or away from the wound edge. The CE, FS, P, PS, PRE, and SBE are reverse cutting needles. Round needles are used to sew fascia.

Needle selection depends on the site being sutured. Different letters designate different series of needles that differ in size, sharpness, and quality.[32] The Ethicon needles, in increasing order of sharpness and quality, are the FS (for skin), PS (plastic skin), P (plastic), CPS (conventional plastic surgery), and PC (precision cosmetic). Davis & Geck's basic needles are the DP (diamond point), CE (cutting 3/8 circle), and SC (skin closure). The PRE (plastic reverse) and SBE (slim blade) are the two higher-quality needles in the series. Needles for skin (FS) and cutting (CE) can be used on the thicker skin of the trunk and extremities. For facial skin, the PC, P, and PRE series are commonly used.

Objective measurements of needle sharpness and deformation have been studied.[33] Comparison of equivalent needles manufactured by Deknatel, Davis & Geck, and Ethicon revealed that Ethicon needles were sharpest and had a decreased propensity to deformation.

Wound Closure Tapes

Wound closure tapes avoid the need to puncture the skin. Tape-closed wounds are more resistant to infection.[34] However, they are rarely used alone in cutaneous surgery because appropriate approximation and eversion is difficult.[26] Skin closure tapes are commonly used to give additional support to the wound after removal of sutures and staples. Compound benzoin tincture or Mastisol (gum mastic, styrax liquid, methyl salicylate, and alcohol) are commonly used to increase adhesiveness. Mastisol's adhesiveness is superior to compound tincture of benzoin.[35] Maximum adhesiveness is obtained after allowing the Mastisol to dry for three minutes. The adhesiveness of all wound closure tapes are enhanced with the use of Mastisol.[36]

Staples

Although disposable and sterilizable models of staplers are available, disposable staplers are most commonly used. Staples are available in regular and wide widths. Regular-width staples are sufficient for all procedures with the exception of scalp reduction.[25] Handling characteristics, ease of positioning, staple-release mechanism, angle of staple delivery, and visibility of staple insertion site should be considered when selecting a stapler.[37] Advantages of staples include rapid wound closure, minimal tissue reaction, and a decreased tendency for wound infection and tissue strangulation. Disadvantages include the cosmetic appearance of staples, and unit cost. Procedures in which staples may be advantageous include split-thickness graft attachment, scalp reduction, wounds closed under a high degree of tension, and axillary vault excisions. Staple extractors ease staple removal.

HEMOSTATIC AGENTS

Introduction

Hemostatic agents used to control small-vessel bleeding can be categorized as mechanical, thermal, topical, and injectable types. Mechanical means of hemostasis are based on the use of pressure either at the site of bleeding or at the edge of the wound. Means of obtaining hemostasis by direct pressure include the use of one's digit, cotton swabs, plastic rings, and instruments such as a chalazion clamp. Thermal hemostasis utilizes heat. Topical and injectable agents including caustic, meshwork, and material. Physiologic agents are available for control of small-vessel bleeding.

Caustic Agents

Monsel's solution (20% ferric sulfate) and aluminum chloride are inexpensive styptics that are easily stored.[38,39] The metal ions of these agents help achieve hemostasis by protein precipitation. The acidity of the solutions may play a role as well.[40] Aluminum chloride is commonly available in concentrations of 20, 35, 50, and 70% solutions in alcohol or water. Monsel's solution is more effective, but causes more tissue damage than aluminum chloride and can uncommonly cause skin hyperpigmentation. Silver nitrate sticks and dichloroacetic or trichloroacetic agents are hemostatic agents that form a zone of eschar. Because these agents damage normal tissue, they are not commonly used for hemostasis.

Meshwork Agents

Absorbable hemostatic agents work by forming an artificial clot or a meshwork that promotes clotting. These agents include absorbable gelatin (Gelfoam), oxidized cellulose (Surgicel, Oxycel), and collagen (Avitene, Collastat, Hemopad, Instat).

Gelfoam is derived from animal gelatin and is available in various-sized sponges or powder forms. Gelfoam has no intrinsic hemostatic action. Because it absorbs 45 times its weight in blood, the pressure of the engorged sponge on the wound results in mechanical hemostasis.[41] In addition, its porous meshwork provides an environment for clot formation.[38] The sponge can be applied dry or moistened with saline or thrombin. Gelfoam is completely absorbed in four to six weeks. Because it is nonantigenic, little tissue reaction is noted.

Oxidized cellulose (Oxycel, Surgicel) is derived from cellulose. Surgicel is available as strips of fabric. Oxycel is available as pads, pledgets, or strips. These products are applied dry to the wound surface and provide a meshwork for clot formation. The material is less irritating to tissue than Gelfoam.[38] Owing to its bactericidal properties, the chance of infection with cellulose is lower than with other similar agents. The material is absorbed within six weeks.[41] This agent should be considered in patients more prone to infections.

Collagen (Hemopad, Helistat, Hemotene, Instat, Collastat sponge, Avitene) is derived from bovine collagen protein. The helical structure of the molecule is responsible for its hemostatic properties.[42] It is available in a fibrillar and microfibrillar form. The material is absorbed within 7–10 weeks. Collagen is more expensive yet more effective as a single agent than cellulose or gelatin,[41] and can be easily removed from the wound. The microfibrillar form should be handled with forceps because it adheres to wet surfaces such as gloves, instruments, and tissue.

Physiologic Agents

Physiologic agents useful in controlling hemostasis are thrombin, epinephrine, and cocaine. Thrombin (Thrombostat, Thrombinar, Thrombogen) is derived from bovine prothrombin protein, which converts fibrinogen to fibrin. Although it can be used in its original freeze-dried powder form, it is most commonly diluted with isotonic saline to a concentration of 100 units per milliliter in cutaneous wounds. Higher concentrations (up to 1000–2000 U/mL) may be needed for profuse bleeding. Because it is absorbed immediately, thrombin is not associated with an increased incidence of infection or foreign-body reactions as is the case with meshwork agents. If thrombin enters a large vessel, thrombosis and death can occur.[42] In contrast to the meshwork agents, thrombin can be used in a wound that will be grafted.

Epinephrine is an alpha adrenergic receptor agonist that promotes vasoconstriction. Both topical and injectable routes may be utilized. Concentrations from 1:1000 to 1:1000000 have been used effectively.[43,44] Although a solution of 1:500000 of epinephrine in lidocaine is effective for hemostasis, these solutions are not stable on a long-term basis.[45] The danger of toxicity from systemic absorption warrants a cautious approach to epinephrine use.

Cocaine is an excellent topical anesthetic for mucous membranes and is a potent vasoconstrictor. Adverse effects include central nervous system stimulation, bradycardia, tachycardia, and hypertension. The medication must be stored in a secure fashion, and careful documentation of its use is required.

Fibrin sealant (fibrin glue, fibrin adhesive, fibrin tissue adhesive) consists of a mixture of concentrated fibrinogen, Factor XIII aprotinin, and fibrinolysis inhibitor, with bovine thrombin and calcium chloride. The mixture of equal amounts of fibrinogen and thrombin result in fibrin clot formation in 30 seconds.[43] Because human plasma is used, there is some risk for bloodborne transmission of infection. Only extemporaneously prepared solutions are available in the United States.[46]

Hydrogen peroxide is mildly hemostatic as a 3% solution. Hydrogen peroxide's primary use is as an aid to wound débridement, achieved by its bubbling action.

ELECTROSURGERY

Electrosurgery utilizes electrically generated thermal energy to achieve hemostasis. Hemostasis can be achieved with electrocautery, electrodesiccation, and electrocoagulation.

Electrocautery usually consists of a direct-current, high-voltage, low-amperage system in which the electric current heats a filament. The filament transfers the heat to the tissue, resulting in protein denaturation and tissue coagulation.[47] Electrocautery units are available in disposable and nondisposable types. Electrocautery is useful in situations in which transfer of electrical current to the patient is not desirable, such as in patients with pacemakers or implantable defibrillators. These units are useful in periorbital surgery when the orbital septum is exposed in order to prevent conduction of electric current into the eye. These units are not extremely effective in a vigorously bleeding field. The Shaw scalpel consists of a scalpel blade that can be heated to temperatures between 110 and 270°C in 10-degree increments.[48] This device allows for simultaneous cutting of tissue and hemostatic control of small and medium-sized vessels. Some dermatologic surgeons find this a useful time-saving device in highly vascularized areas.

Electrocoagulation and electrodesiccation differ in the method of current delivery.[49] Electrodesiccation consists of a high-voltage, high-frequency, low-amperage current. This results in desiccation of tissue. Electrocoagulation is a high-frequency current that is lower in voltage and higher in amperage than electrodesiccation. Electrocoagulation is more effective in stopping actively bleeding vessels.

Various accessories are available with electrosurgical devices. These include pencils that allow for fingertip control in activating the current as well as adjustment of the power settings. Alternatively, foot switches can be used to activate the current. Electrodes may be disposable or reusable as well as sterile and nonsterile.[50] Furthermore, various size and shape electrodes are available. Most electrodes are monopolar: there is one single treatment electrode. The most common monopolar electrodes are the needle, ball, and wire electrodes.[47,50,51] Electrodes should not be reused between patients owing to the possibility of bacterial and viral transmission.[52,53]

The sterility of the surgical field can be maintained by covering the electrosurgical handle and cord with a sterile Penrose drain or specifically designed plastic sleeves.[54] Some models have reusable handles and cords that can be resterilized. Others have disposable sterilized handles and cords.

Electrosurgical units may be placed on carts that allow for movement from room to room. In addition, it also offers mobility within the room in order to access any area on the patient. Wall-mounted systems allow for conservation of floor space.

The dispersive electrode, also referred to as the ground plate, indifferent electrode, or return electrode, is used with many electrosurgery units. Current is directed via the dispersive plate back to the electrosurgical unit. Therefore, it prevents the possible exit of current through an alternative route, which may result in an electrical shock or burn to the patient or surgeon. The flat metal plate is the most popular dispersive electrode used in dermatologic surgery. Disposable adhesive dispersive electrodes, which can be applied to nondependent surfaces, provide the greatest degree of safety. The patient should not be in contact with any metal surfaces on the examination table.

SMOKE EVACUATORS

The potential hazards of the plume liberated from electrosurgery include the smoke particulate themselves and the potential aerosolization of infectious particles such as papillomavirus, hepatitis B virus, and human immunodeficiency virus.[55] Electrocautery smoke generated in the treatment of 1 g of canine tongue was shown to be mutagenic in *Salmonella typhimurium* strains and equivalent to three to six cigarettes.[56] Although infectious bovine papillomavirus and human papillomavirus DNA have been isolated from warts treated with electrocoagulation, there have not been numerous anecdotal reports documenting infection.[57] When compared to carbon dioxide laser plume, electrosurgical plume is less dense, and less virus is recovered.[58] Surgical masks effectively filtered almost all papillomavirus. No evidence is available regarding the presence or infectiousness of other viruses in electrocautery plume. Until such data are available it would be prudent to adopt safety recommendations formulated for laser plume entailing the use of surgical masks, protective gowns, eye protection, and smoke evacuator systems. The smoke evacuator should be placed no more than 5 cm from the operative site.[59] Other parameters that may affect emission collection include smoke evacuator flow rate, the angle of the nozzle in relation to external air flow, and nozzle configuration.[60]

Factors to consider in selecting a smoke evacuator include the noise during operation of the device, mobility, hose length, filtration efficiency, air flow speed, and replacement cost of filters.

STOCK SUPPLIES

Surgical Gloves

Universal precautions dictate that sterile or nonsterile gloves should be used for situations in which there is potential for contact with human body fluid. Surgical glove perforation was noted in 11.7% of single gloves in a dermatologic surgery clinic.[61] A study of double gloving showed no case of perforation in both the outer and inner gloves on the same hand.[62] Therefore, double gloving may offer an additional protection to the surgeon and patient. These studies do not account for known needle puncture, which may result in a higher infection rate.[63] Cut-resistant protective liners are available to be worn under surgical gloves. Latex gloves are less likely to have leaks than vinyl gloves.[64] The health care worker should recognize that no glove is foolproof, and that hand washing should be performed after removal of gloves.

Patients and health care workers may be allergic to various components of gloves.[65] Recently, latex allergy with clinical manifestations ranging from urticaria to anaphylaxis has been a cause of concern. Hypoallergenic gloves can contain latex protein.[66,67] Vinyl, synthetic neoprene, or tactylon gloves should be substituted in instances of latex allergy.[67]

Needles and Syringes

Syringes are available in disposable and reusable forms. The Luer lock feature allows for high-pressure injection without fear of blowing off the needle and spraying the patient, physician, or staff. Tuberculin syringes are useful for postoperative injection of corticosteroids into flaps. The 3-mm syringe is useful for anesthesia infiltration in biopsies. The three-ring syringe aids in the delivery of larger volumes of anesthesia for excisions. Syringes with protective sheath locks afford additional protection against accidental needle sticks. The most commonly used needle are the 30-gauge needles. Twenty-five gauge needles are useful for corticosteroid injection of flaps. Smaller 32- and 33-gauge microneedles in various lengths are available for sclerotherapy.

Protective Clothes

Protective gowns, masks, and eye shields are needed for adequate protection in dermatologic surgery and to satisfy OSHA requirements. Disposable gowns are most convenient for the non-hospital-based surgeon. Masks are available with clear plastic eyeshields. Alternatively, separate eye and face shields are available.

Surgical Drapes

Surgical drapes are available in reusable cloth and disposable paper forms. For the office-based practice paper drapes may be more convenient. Since implementation of OSHA's Bloodborne Pathogens Standard, a wide array of personal protective equipment is available. Cloth drapes conform better to the patient and are more easily stabilized than paper drapes.

CONCLUSION

The setting up of a surgical facility requires attention to many details relating to the physical plant and equipment. A knowledge and understanding of the factors that play a role in the selection and design of equipment facilitates the decisions necessary to customize a surgical practice. This foundation allows the physician to select equipment rather than limit his choices to his training experiences.

REFERENCES

1. Tobin HA. Office surgery: The surgical suite. *J Dermatol Surg Oncol.* 14:247–255, 1988.
2. Maloney ME. *The Dermatologic Surgical Suite: Design and Materials.* New York, NY: Churchill Livingstone; 1991.
3. Bennett RG. *Fundamentals of Cutaneous Surgery.* St Louis, MO: CV Mosby; 1988, pp 181–193, 784–789.
4. Dermatology Practice Administration: OSHA hazard communication. American Academy of Dermatology, 1993.
5. Dermatology Practice Administration: Bloodborne pathogens. American Academy of Dermatology, 1992.
6. Sebben JE. Surgical antiseptics. *J Am Acad Dermatol.* 9:759–765, 1983.
7. Laufman H. Current use of skin and wound cleansers and antiseptics. *Am J Surg* 175:359–365, 1989.
8. Dzubow LM, Halpern AC, Leyden JJ, et al. Comparison of preoperative skin preparations for the face. *J Am Acad Dermatol* 19:737–741, 1988.
9. Howard RJ. Surgical infections. In: Schwartz SI, Shires GT, Spencer, FC. *Principles of Surgery,* 6th ed. New York, NY: McGraw Hill; 1994; 145.
10. Takegami KT, Siegle RJ, Ayers LW. Microbiologic counts during outpatient office-based cutaneous surgery. *J Am Acad Dermatol* 23:1149–1152, 1990.
11. Siegel DM. A new scalpel handle for the cutaneous surgeon. *J Dermatol Surg Oncol.* 1989; 15:1251.
12. Bernstein G: The 15c scalpel blade. *J Dermatol Surg Oncol.* 13:969, 1987.
13. Robinson JK. Excision of benign pigmented nevi by shave technique. *J Dermatol Surg Oncol.* 6:166, 1980.

14. Sebben JE. Surgical instruments and the cutaneous surgery practice, 3rd ed. Focus Session, Annual Meeting American Academy of Dermatology, Washington, DC 1988.

15. Grabski WJ, SJ Salasche, MJ Mulvaney. Razor-blade surgery. *J Dermatol Surg Oncol.* 16:1121–1126, 1990.

16. Grande DJ, Neuburg M. Instrumentation for the dermatologic surgeon. *J Dermatol Surg Oncol.* 15:288–297, 1989.

17. Frankel DH. The use of a combination skin hook and tissue forceps: A new instrument for dermatologic surgery ("Frankel-Adson Forceps"). *J Dermatol Surg Oncol.* 14:497–499, 1988.

18. Lerner SP. The modified skin hook: A new instrument in cutaneous surgery. *J Dermatol Oncol.* 11:586–588, 1985.

19. Robinson JK. Some tips on wound closure. *J Dermatol Surg Oncol.* 8:698–700, 1982.

20. Bernstein G: The Castroviejo needle holder. *J Dermatol Surg Oncol.* 14:21–22, 1988.

21. Sebben JE. Sterile technique and the prevention of wound infection in office surgery-part I. *J Dermatol Surg Oncol.* 14:1364–1371, 1988.

22. Sebben JE. Sterilization and care of surgical instruments and supplies. *J Am Acad Dermatol.* 11:381–392, 1984.

23. Klapes NA, Greene VW, Langholz AC, et al. Effect of long-term storage on sterile status of devices in surgical packs. *Infect Control.* 8:289–293, 1987.

24. Pollock SV. Rapid instrument sterilization. *J Dermatol Surg Oncol.* 16:438–439, 1990.

25. Bennett RG. Selection of wound closure materials. *J Am Acad Dermatol.* 18:619–637, 1988.

26. Moy RL, Walman B, Hein DW. A review of sutures and suturing techniques. *J Dermatol Surg Oncol.* 18:785–795, 1992.

27. Brunius U, Zederfeldt B. Suture materials in general surgery: A comment. *Prog Surg.* 8:38–44, 1970.

28. Webster RC, McCollough EG, Giandello PR, et al. Skin wound approximation with new absorbable suture material. *Arch Otolaryngol.* 111:517–519, 1985.

29. Ray JA, Doddi N, Regula D, et al. Polydioxanone (PDS), a novel monofilament synthetic absorbable suture. *Surg Gynecol Obstet.* 153:497–503, 1981.

30. Katz AR, Mukherjee DP, Kaganov AL, et al. A new synthetic monofilament absorbable suture made from polytrimethylene carbonate. *Surg Gynecol Obstet.* 161:213–222, 1985.

31. Moy RM, Kaufman AJ. Clinical comparison of polyglactic acid (vicryl) and polytrimethylene carbonate (Maxon) suture material. *J Dermatol Surg Oncol.* 17:667–669; 1991.

32. Garrett AB: Wound closure materials. In: Wheeland RG. *Cutaneous Surgery.* Philadelphia, PA: WB Saunders; 1994:199.

33. Edlich RF, Towler MA, Rodeheaver GT et al. Scientific basis for selecting surgical needles and needle holders for wound closure. *Clin Plast Surg.* 17:583–602, 1990.

34. Edlich RF, Becker DG, Thacker JG, et al. Scientific basis for selecting staple and tape skin closures. *Clin Plast Surg.* 17:571–581, 1990.

35. Mikhail GR, Selak L, Salo S. Reinforcement of surgical adhesive strips. *J Dermatol Surg Oncol.* 12:904–906, 1986.

36. Moy RL, Quan MB. An evaluation of wound closure tapes. *J Dermatol Surg Oncol.* 16:721–723, 1990.

37. Campbell JP, Swanson NA. The use of staples in dermatologic surgery. *J Dermatol Surg Oncol.* 8:680–690, 1982.

38. Dinehart S. How to stop bleeding in dermatologic surgery. Focus session, Annual Meeting American Academy of Dermatology, Washington, DC 1993.

39. Epstein E. Topical hemostatic agents for dermatologic surgery. J Dermatol Surg Oncol. 15:342–343, 1989.

40. Larson PO. Dr. Larson replies. *J Dermatol Surg Oncol.* 1989; 15:343.

41. Arand AG, Sawaya R. Intraoperative chemical hemostasis in neurosurgery. *Neurosurgery.* 18:223–233, 1986.

42. American Medical Association, Hemostatics, in *Drug Evaluation Annual 1993*. Chicago, 1993:785.

43. Larson PO. Topical hemostatic agents for dermatologic surgery. *J Dermatol Surg Oncol.* 14:623–632, 1988.

44. Siegel RJ, Vistne LM, Iverson RE. Effective hemostasis with less epinephrine. *Plast Reconst Surg.* 51:129–133, 1973.

45. Grabb WC. A concentration of 1:500,000 epinephrine in a local anesthetic solution is sufficient to provide excellent hemostasis. *Plast Reconst Surg.* 63:834, 1979.

46. Thompson DF, Letassy NA, Thompson GD. Fibrin glue: A review of its preparation, efficacy, and adverse effects as a topical hemostat. *Drug Intell Clin Pharm.* 22:946–952, 1988.

47. Sebben JE. *Cutaneous Electrosurgery*. Chicago, IL: Year Book Medical Publishers; 1989 pp 5–25.

48. Tromovitch TA, Glogau RG, Stegman SJ. The Shaw scalpel. *J Dermatol Surg Oncol.* 9:316–319, 1983.

49. Sebben JE. Contamination risks associated with electrosurgery. *Arch Dermatol.* 126:805–807, 1990.

50. Sebben JE. Modifications of electrosurgery electrodes. *J Dermatol Surg Oncol.* 18:908–912, 1992.

51. Pollack SV. *Electrosurgery of the Skin*. New York, NY: Churchill Livingstone; 1991 pp 7–20.

52. Bennett RG, Kraffert CA. Bacterial transference during electrodesiccation and electrocoagulation. *Arch Dermatol.* 126:751–755, 1990.

53. Sherertz EF, Davis GL, Rice RW, et al. Transfer of hepatitis B virus by contaminated reusable needle electrodes after electrodesiccation in simulated use. *J Am Acad Dermatol.* 15:1242–1246, 1986.

54. Stoner JG, Swanson NA, Vargo N. Penrose sleeve. *J Dermatol Surg Oncol.* 9:523–524, 1983.

55. Berberian BJ, Burnett JW. The potential role of common dermatologic practice technics in transmitting disease. *J Am Acad Dermatol.* 15:1057–1058, 1986.

56. Tomita Y, Mihashi S, Nagata K, et al. Mutagenicity of smoke condensates induced by CO_2 laser irradiation and electrocauterization. *Mutat Res.* 89:145–149, 1989.

57. Sawchuck WS, Felton RP. Infectious potential of aerosolized particles. *Arch Dermatol.* 125:1689–1692, 1989.

58. Sawchuck WS, Weber PJ, Lowy DR, et al. Infectious papillomavirus in the vapor of warts treated with carbon dioxide laser or electrocoagulation: detection and protection. *J Am Acad Dermatol.* 21:41–49, 1989.

59. Smith JP, Moss CE, Bryant CJ, et al. Evaluation of a smoke evacuator used for laser surgery. *Lasers Surg Med.* 9:276–281, 1981.

60. Smith JP, Topmiller JL, Shulman S. Factors affecting emission collection by surgical smoke evacuators. *Lasers Surg Med.* 10:224–233, 1990.

61. Gross DJ, Jamison Y, Martin K, et al. Surgical glove perforation in dermatologic surgery. *J Dermatol Surg Oncol.* 15:1226–1228, 1989.

62. Cohen MS, Do JT, Tahery DP, et al. Efficacy of double gloving as a protection against blood exposure in dermatologic surgery. *J Dermatol Surg Oncol.* 18:873–874, 1992.

63. Robinson JK. Safety issues, risks, and precautions for dermatologic surgery. *Cutis.* 52:345–347, 1993.

64. Olsen RJ, Lynch P, Coyle MB, et al. Examination gloves as barriers to hand contamination in clinical practice. *JAMA.* 270:350–353, 1993.

65. Maso MJ, Goldberg DJ. Contact dermatoses from disposable glove use: A review. *J Am Acad Dermatol.* 23:733–737, 1990.

66. Wolf BL. Anaphylactic reaction to latex gloves. *N Engl J Med.* 329:279–280, 1993.

67. Taylor JS. Latex allergy. *Am J Contact Dermatitis.* 4:114–117, 1993.

4

PLANNING THE EXCISION

J. Greg Brady, DO

Terry L. Barrett, MD

To ensure the best result in the excision of a problematic benign or malignant lesion, preoperative planning and patient counseling must be done even for the most minor procedure. It is important that the patient understand the need for the surgery and that a scar will result from any biopsy or excisional surgery. Although timeliness may be important in some cases, there are no emergency excisions. There is plenty of time to plan carefully, consult reference material, and elicit the advice and help of physicians in other specialities if needed.

PREOPERATIVE DIAGNOSIS

Clinical Exam

Determine the location and extent of the lesion within the skin. The clinical margin is defined as the junction of the lesion with normal skin. Cleansing the area with an alcohol pad, stretching the skin, magnification, good lighting, side lighting, palpation, epilumescence microscopy, Woods' lighting of pigmented lesions, and transillu-

---

*The opinions or assertions contained herein are the private views of the authors and are not to be construed as official or as reflecting the views of the Department of the Navy or the Department of Defense.

mination of cystic lesions all may assist in making an accurate determination of the clinical margin of the lesion. In most cases the depth or extent of the lesion can be placed within one or more of the following layers: epidermis, dermis, subcutaneous fat, fascia, muscle, periosteum or bone. The purpose of a biopsy is to obtain a representative sample of the lesion. The biopsy must be deep and wide enough to contain adequate tissue to reflect accurately the lesion's cellular makeup and architecture. With generalized lesions multiple biopsies may be required to gain an adequate sampling of the pathology. Effective management of cutaneous malignant neoplasms may require that regional lymph nodes be carefully inspected before surgery. This is of particular concern with squamous cell carcinoma and malignant melanoma, as local measures alone will be ineffective in cases with regional or systemic spread. Lymph nodes may enlarge for a short time postoperatively secondary to inflammation from the surgical procedure, giving the false appearance of regional spread.

Lesions may occupy one or more levels in the skin although they tend to originate from only one level (Figure 4-1). Hyperkeratosis, ulceration, vesiculation, and pigmentation are features of an epidermal lesion. A firm raised nodule or plaque that moves easily with the skin is characteristic of a dermal lesion. Lesions located in the subcutaneous fat tend to be more diffuse in nature, lack sharp margins, and are usually larger than the clinical estimate. Subcutaneous lesions may be movable or fixed to the layer above or below. Lesions of the fascia are relatively immobile, and the skin can usually be moved over the lesion. The size of a lesion at or below the level of the fascia is very difficult to estimate by palpation. Prior to biopsy, imaging studies (x-ray, CAT scan, MRI, and/or Ultrasound) should be considered for lesions located in the midline of the scalp.[1-5] Lesions that move with the underlying muscle or are fixed to the fascia or bone usually require regional or general anesthesia for resection, and consultation with other specialties may be needed.

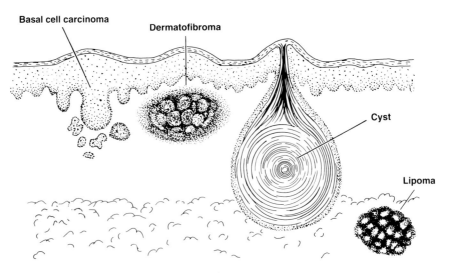

Figure 4.1. The type of biopsy needed corresponds to the location of the lesion within the skin.

Documenting Location

It is essential that documentation such as an accurate map be drawn of the location of the lesion before biopsy (Figure 4-2). Shave biopsies can heal with an almost imperceptible scar. It is uncomfortable and distressing to both patient and physician when a search must be undertaken to find the biopsy site. It is even more distressing when the physician operates on the wrong site, mistaking an area of erythema for a previous biopsy site. Shave biopsies that saucerize the lesion or take a vertical wedge from the center of the lesion tend to heal with a depressed scar marking the site. Punch biopsies have the advantage that the patient must return for suture removal and will have sutures marking the biopsy site. A delay in definitive treatment for three to four weeks can even make a punch biopsy site barely visible, especially in a patient with severe actinic damage. Therefore, it is essential that the physician use a method that allows the site of the biopsy to be located again with confidence.

The map may be from stencil, paste on diagrams, anatomic rubber stamp, or full-page diagrams.[6] Full-page diagrams can be made using a copier to enlarge any of the smaller diagrams you may be using. Larger-sized diagrams allow you to accurately and precisely pinpoint the lesion using distances from two or three surface landmarks or fixed bony prominences as reference points.

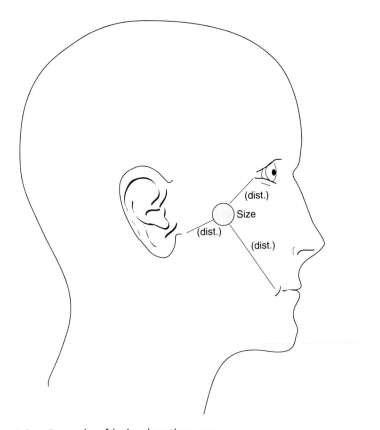

Figure 4.2.   Example of lesion location map.

A more costly but very accurate technique is the use of photography to document the location of lesions. Flesh-colored or poorly defined lesions may need to be outlined using a skin marker before taking the photograph. Polaroid photographs (cost/photo) are more expensive than 35-mm slides but have the advantage of being available for immediate review and placement in the patient's chart. Slides and photographs using a 35-mm format provide sharp images and accurately document lesion location and morphology. An office video camera and recorder could also be used to document the preoperative location of lesions. Newer techniques using digital imaging are still very expensive for office use but may become more affordable as the technology becomes more prevalent.

In patients with severe actinic damage or in areas where there are few landmarks, a tattoo can be placed at the site of the biopsy using a drop of india ink and a needle. We recommend this technique only after the pathology is known and it has been determined that the area must be reexcised, as the tattoo will be permanent.

PATIENT EVALUATION

Focused History and Physical

The physician must be aware of any medical condition or medication that could adversely affect the outcome of a biopsy or excision. A focused history and physical exam should be completed before any surgical procedure, as even a minor procedure can have untoward results.

The history should include allergies to topical and systemic medications, with specific questioning on medications or dressings to be used during or following surgery (ie, providone-iodine, lidocaine, bacitracin, and surgical tape), consider the possible drug interactions that may occur during surgery, and present medications including aspirin and nonsteroidal anti-inflammatory use.[7] Aspirin is in many OTC medications as well as Chinese vitamins, and the patient may be unaware of taking it unless specifically asked. A current listing of aspirin-containing compounds can be found in the *Physicians' Desk Reference Generic* and *Chemical Name Index* under "aspirin." Some of the more common medications that contain occult aspirin are Alka-Seltzer, Anacin, Ascriptin, Bufferin, 4-Way Cold Tablets, Fiorinal, Norgesic, Percodan, Ecotrin, and Excedrin Extra-Strength.

The patient should also be questioned about previous surgeries and presence of artificial joints, cardiac pacemaker, heart valves, and keloidal tendencies. Medical conditions that could be affected by a surgical procedure include susceptibility to fainting, pregnancy, high blood pressure, cardiac disease, angina, myocardial infarction, mitral valve prolapse with regurgitation, seizures, diabetes, or infectious diseases that may put the operating team at increased risk, such as hepatitis and HIV.

Personal habits such as smoking and alcohol intake may also compromise the results of a surgical procedure. Flap and graft necrosis is three times higher in high-level smokers (one or more packs per day) than in patients who never smoked, former smokers, or low-level smokers (less than one pack per day).[8]

The physical exam should concentrate on the presence of any motor paralysis, sensory deficit, facial asymmetry, previous surgical scars, concurrent dermatoses at or near the surgical site, regional lymph nodes, bruises, and other lesions in the proximity of the lesion. Note should also be made of anatomic structures that may be altered by removal of the lesion.

It is strongly recommended that a patient questionnaire covering these concerns serve as a preoperative checklist for procedures to avoid errors of omission.

Adaptations in Management Based on the History and Physical

Based on the history and physical examination, the type of biopsy may be modified or delayed to reduce the risk to the patient. Medications may have to be substituted if there are allergies.[9] Preoperative antibiotics may be required depending on site and presence of mitral valve prolapse, artificial heart valves or joint replacement.[10,11] They may also be used two days before and two days after surgery to decrease the incidence of postoperative infections.[12]

We try to postpone excisional surgery on patients for 10 days following the last use of aspirin. Aspirin irreversibly inhibits cyclo-oxygenase for the life of the platelet.[13] This delay in surgery is based on the replacement rate of platelets, as functional platelets are released into the circulation at a rate of approximately 10% per day after aspirin has been discontinued. Ideally we restart aspirin at the time of suture removal. In cases of cardiovascular or cerebrovascular disease, the patient's internist is consulted before discontinuing the aspirin. We also discontinue all nonsteroidal anti-inflammatory drugs six days before surgery. For nonsteroidal medications, the platelet effects are reversible after discontinuance of the medication, so the effects are not as long lasting.

If the surgery will involve the periorbital region, use of chlorhexidine as a surgical skin preparation is strongly discouraged as it is extremely toxic to the cornea and can result in a progressive keratopathy.[14,15]

Monitoring or the use of bipolar forceps or hot cautery may be needed in patients with cardiac pacemakers.[16,17]

Hypertensive episodes coupled with reflex bradycardia and cardiac arrest have occurred even with small doses of epinephrine in patients taking β-blockers, especially with a nonselective β-blocker like propanolol. The minimum amount of epinephrine, 1:200,000, which will provide ample anesthesia and hemostasis, should be used. Consider switching the patient to a selective β-blocker in cases that will require more than a minimal amount of anesthesia, as a cardiac arrest has been reported with as little as 13 mL of 0.5% lidocaine with 1:200,000 epinephrine.[18,19] The concentration of epinephrine may be reduced to 1:200,000 in patients with cardiovascular disease by diluting the stock 1% lidocaine with 1:100,000 epinephrine with an equal amount of 1% lidocaine plain and still obtain effective hemostasis.

In children and severely apprehensive patients, ice, iontophoresis of local anesthesia, or EMLA cream may be used for shave biopsies or before injection to reduce the pain of local anesthesia.[20] To further reduce the pain of infiltration, lidocaine can be buffered with epinephrine by mixing 30 mL of the anesthetic with 3 mL of 8.4% sodium bicarbonate (1 meq/mL).[21] This solution will be stable for two weeks if kept refrigerated at 0–4°C.[22]

Patients who smoke more than two packs per day should stop smoking or reduce their smoking level to below one pack per day 48 hours before the surgery and for a week following the surgery if a flap or graft is contemplated.[9]

BIOPSY

An accurate preoperative diagnosis is essential to planning the surgical removal of a lesion. The margins and depth of a surgical excision should be determined by the biology of the lesion. A dermatologist or other physician with special training or experience can often determine the diagnosis by careful clinical inspection of the lesion morphology and location. In addition to lighting and magnification, epilumescence microscopy has recently been added to the armamentarium to assist with the clinical differential diagnosis.[23–25] However, without a histopathologic diagnosis the surgeon may be too aggressive in the removal of a benign lesion or too conservative with a malignant one.

Histopathologic examination remains the gold standard for determining the exact nature of the lesion. The purpose of the biopsy is to provide an accurate histopathological diagnosis. The surgeon should provide as much information as possible including the size of the lesion and its duration, extent, and differential diagnosis to assist the pathologist in correlation of the histologic findings with the clinical data to arrive at an accurate diagnosis.

Biopsy Options

After determining the clinical margin a decision has to be made whether to perform a biopsy on a portion of the lesion or attempt to perform a complete excision. There are different options for a biopsy depending on the clinical diagnosis, location, and extent of the lesion (see Table 4-1). Shave and punch biopsies are the most commonly performed diagnostic procedures for lesion sampling. They often provide excellent samples for determining the nature of a lesion. The maximum-size punch that one should use is 4 mm. Punch biopsies larger than this will result in a defect that is difficult to close owing to the amount of redundant tissue that forms at the apices when closure is attempted. A fusiform excision is recommended for biopsy of lesions larger than 4 mm.

Shave biopsies and punch biopsies are not recommended on small atypical pigmented lesions. If the lesion is a melanoma, a shave biopsy may not include the base of the lesion, making the determination of the Breslow measurement and Clark's level impossible. These measurements of the depth of invasion of malignant melanoma are the basis on which the proper surgical margin and prognosis are based. A punch biopsy of a small atypical pigmented lesion may have the most critical area inadvertently discarded when the punch is processed (see Punch Biopsy following). An incisional or excisional biopsy may be considered depending on clinical diagnosis, location, and size. If a malignant melanoma is in the differential diagnosis of a pigmented lesion, an excisional biopsy of the entire lesion with a 1-mm surgical margin is our preferred method of biopsy.

Shave Biopsy

Epidermal and superficial dermal lesions may have biopsies performed on them by using a shave technique that removes the epidermis and the papillary dermis. The anes-

Table 4.1.   Recommended Biopsy Techniques for Selected Lesions

Shave Biopsy:	Benign nevi
	Pyogenic granuloma
	Skin tags
	Epidermal tumors
	Verruca
	Seborrheic keratoses
	Molluscum
Punch Biopsy:	Epidermal tumors
	Inflammatory lesions
	Generalized dermatoses
	Granulomas
	Infectious lesions (histology and culture)
	Dermal tumors
	Tumors of the epidermal appendages
	Metabolic diseases
Incisional Biopsy:	Large pigmented lesions
	Lesions with transition areas
	(morphea and porokeratosis)
	Inflammatory lesions of the fat or fascia
	(erythema nodosum and eosinophilic fasciitis)
Excisional Biopsy:	Atypical melanocytic lesions
	Nevi with hair or deep pigmentation
	Epidermal/pilar cysts
	Fibrous tissue tumors
	Tumors of the fat
	Dermal nevi
	Metastatic lesions

thetic can be used to raise the area so that a horizontal shave will remove a saucerized specimen. Suspected benign lesions may be shaved superficially. However, suspected basal cell carcinoma (BCC) and squamous cell carcinoma (SCC) should be shaved deeper to include the majority of the base of the lesion. This technique is not recommended for the sampling of recurrent lesions or those suspected of being infiltrative or morpheaform basal cell carcinomas.

The shave biopsy site tends to heal with a flat or slightly depressed scar. The amount of depression depends on the depth of the shave. The depth of the damage is increased through chemical cautery using 35% aluminum chloride (Drysol) or ferric sulfate (Monsel's), both of which produce tissue necrosis by denaturing protein.[26,27] Ferric sulfate carries the additional risk of iron staining of the biopsy site. A hyfercator can also be used to control bleeding. Additionally, hemostasis can be obtained by using direct pressure, an absorbable gelatin sponge, oxidized regenerated cellulose, micronized collagen, or thrombin. These alternate methods should be considered in situations where minimal scar formation is important.

Punch Biopsy

Epidermal and dermal lesions may have biopsies performed on them by using a punch biopsy. This biopsy technique is a quick and useful way to obtain a portion of a large lesion or representative samples of a generalized dermatitis. A 3- or 4-mm punch biopsy is adequate for sampling most lesions. Punch biopsy sites are usually sutured closed for hemostasis and cosmesis. However, they do not have to be sutured closed, as gelatin foam may be placed in the defect for hemostasis. The final cosmetic result may be similar using either approach. The use of gelatin foam instead of suturing has proved useful in minimizing the exposure of operating personnel to sharps.

Punch biopsies should not be used on suspected BCC or SCC that will be treated using electrodessication and curettage. As a punch normally goes completely through the dermis to the subcutaneous fat, it disrupts the dermis. An intact dermis is the keystone for utilizing the curette to define the extent of the tumor.

As previously stated, punch biopsies are not advised for obtaining a specimen of small atypical pigmented lesions or for lesions that require clear surgical margins. It is almost impossible for the pathologist to orient the specimen and obtain margins histologically. Just "getting around" a malignant tumor with a punch is inadequate treatment. Although it is recommended that 4-mm punch biopsies be processed in toto, it is common practice for the pathologist to bisect a punch biopsy that is 4 mm or larger to enhance processing of the tissue.[28] After the tissue is bisected, the cut edge is positioned in the tissue cassette such that this edge will be sectioned first on the microtome. The histology technician then faces (cuts) the block to get a complete section. In this facing process the technician may cut away and discard many incomplete sections from the central, most important portion of the lesion. This central portion is exactly the point on which most clinicians center their punch when taking the biopsy (Figure 4-3).

Punch biopsies are helpful on very large pigmented lesions that have ample areas of pathology for the purpose of sampling portions of the lesion and in cases where an excisional or fusiform incisional biopsy is not possible. Imbedding in toto and stepping the block rather than bisecting the tissue may be recommended in these cases. The clinician must request that the specimen be processed in this manner at the time it is submitted to pathology. Punch biopsy specimens 5 mm or larger, because of technical considerations, must be bisected for adequate fixation and processing. Therefore, the use of 5-mm or larger punch biopsies should be limited.

Incisional Biopsy

Performing a biopsy on a portion of a large lesion in a fusiform manner yields more tissue for diagnosis and evaluation of architecture. The fusiform sampling may be taken through the center or most atypical portion of a lesion, or may be oriented to sample the transition zone between involved and normal tissue, which can aid in the diagnosis of processes such as morphea.

A vertical wedge biopsy is used by some practitioners as a variation of the horizontal shave technique to take a sample of a suspected basal cell carcinoma or squamous cell carcinoma within the peripheral confines of the margin of the tumor.[29] This technique preserves the peripheral tumor margin and may be helpful in allowing one to find the biopsy site of a BCC or SCC in a severely sun-damaged patient at a later time.

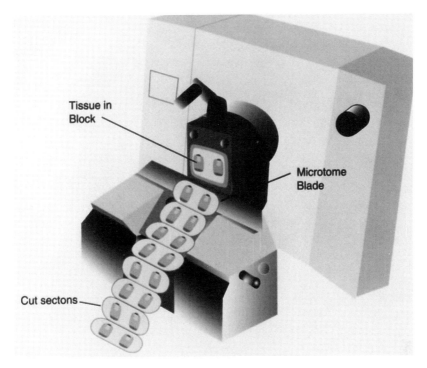

Tissue in
Block

Microtome
Blade

Cut sectons

Figure 4.3. Facing the block. A portion of the specimen is actually cut
away and discarded to obtain a complete section for histologic examination.

Excisional Biopsy

An excisional biopsy is used on lesions that involve multiple layers of the skin or
are located deeper than the epidermal layer. Excisional surgery involves taking a border of normal skin beyond the clinical margin to completely remove the lesion. This is
called the surgical margin (see Figure 4-4).

We have found that an excisional biopsy to the subcutaneous fat with a 1-mm surgical margin is adequate to yield an accurate pathologic diagnosis and, in most cases,
will completely remove most benign lesions that involve the epidermis and dermis.
This 1-mm surgical margin is frequently inadequate for treatment of malignant lesions,
and further surgery may be required.

The excisional biopsy specimen should be tagged for orientation using a single
simple suture placed at one of the tips of the specimen. We recommend that the tag of
suture be placed before complete removal of the specimen to ensure accurate orientation. Orientation can easily be lost if the surgeon must attend to hemostasis and places
the unmarked specimen on the tray. The suture tag should be placed after the specimen
has been completely separated at the peripheral margin and is an island of tissue sitting
on the subcutaneous fat. The location of this tag superior, inferior, medial, lateral, or
based on a clock face should be noted in the patient's chart and on the tissue exam

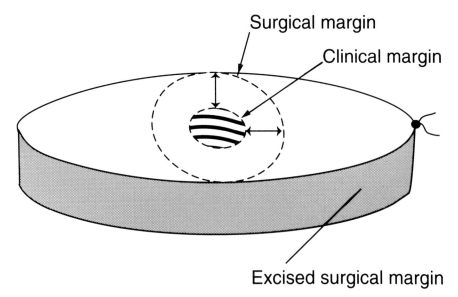

Figure 4.4. Fusiform excisional biopsy showing the location of the lesion, clinical margin, surgical margin, and excised surgical margin.

request form. This allows the pathologist to orient the specimen based on the patient and gives a more accurate interpretation of the examined lateral and deep excised surgical margins.

It is possible to use a modified excisional technique to obtain a complete sample of a small lesion instead of using a punch biopsy.[30] A #11 blade on a blade handle, oriented perpendicular to the skin, is used like a jigsaw to excise a fusiform shape around the lesion with a 1-mm surgical margin. Small up-and-down strokes are made with the #11 blade, the tip just passing into the subcutaneous fat. The specimen obtained can be tagged for orientation, and the wound is easily approximated with sutures. This technique has been especially useful in the biopsy of bullous lesions, allowing the biopsy to be taken with minimal disruption of the epidermis. It is also useful for lesions 3 to 6 mm in diameter and in areas of thicker, less elastic skin and scar tissue, both of which are difficult to approximate when a punch biopsy is used because of the formation of redundant tissue at the apices (see Figure 4-5).

EXCISION DESIGN

Excisions are usually fusiform. The typical length-to-width ratio should be 3:1 to 4:1 with the apical angles measuring 30 degrees, depending on the elasticity of the skin at the site. The long axis is oriented along relaxed skin tension lines or within cosmetic junctions.[31] The skin tension lines may be influenced by positioning, and it is recommended that patients, particularly older ones, be evaluated in a seated or standing position. Also, the skin tension lines are oriented more vertically when the patient is in a

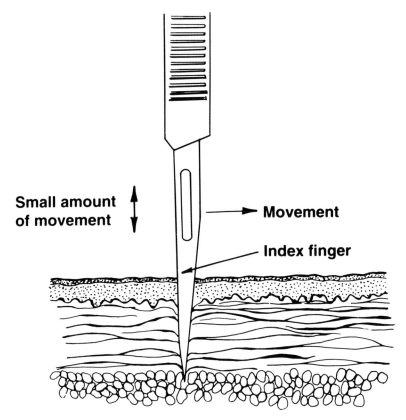

Figure 4.5.   Modified excisional technique utilizing a #11 blade. Small up-and-down strokes of approximately 3 mm are used so that the tip of the blade is just within the subcutaneous tissue. A fusiform shape is excised moving the blade forward like a jigsaw.

sitting or standing position; it is in this position that the patient spends the majority of time.[32] Prior to administering local anesthesia, it is helpful to cleanse the area with alcohol. Then a skin marker is used to draw a few of the skin tension lines that pass near or through the lesion, which assists with orientation while the patient is in a vertical position. Removal of malignant lesions in a fusiform shape maximizes the excised surgical margin in all aspects, except for one section of the lateral margins, and results in minimal rearrangement of tissue (Figure 4-6).

Outlining the Surgical Margin

Drawing the clinical margin of the lesion, then drawing the required surgical margin around the lesion gives one a good idea of the width of the excision needed. This allows an estimation of the adequacy of adjacent tissue required for closure. The fusiform shape should be drawn around the recommended surgical margin with the proper length-to-width ratio and orientation. This helps both the surgeon and the

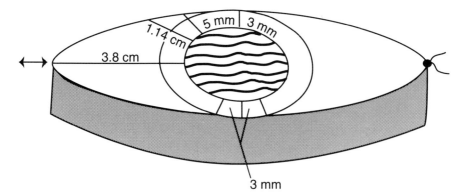

Figure 4.6. Fusiform excision showing representative surgical margins. In this example, the desired surgical margin is 3 mm. However, as can be seen, in most directions, the actual surgical margin is substantially more than 3 mm. The fusiform is oriented along skin tension lines.

patient obtain a realistic image of the actual amount of tissue that will be removed, anatomic danger areas that the excision may cross, and length of the scar. Lesions always seem larger after the patient is prepped, anesthetized, and on the operating table. Patients often underestimate the length of the scar that will result from the removal of what they consider to be a small lesion. Showing them the outlined excision site before performing the surgery will help make their estimate more realistic.

Modifications of the Fusiform Excision

Age Factors

The suggested angles of the apices of a fusiform excision may be increased from a 30-degree angle to a 60-degree angle in older patients and may be decreased from a 30-degree angle to a 20-degree angle in younger patients, depending on the elasticity of the tissue.

Length

A fusiform excision can be lengthened to correct for redundant tissue at the apices. It is preferable to lengthen the wound early in the wound closure if required to allow access to the area for hemostasis and undermining rather than waiting until most of the sutures have been placed. The wound lengthening can be attained through standard standing cone (dog ear) repair, M-plasty, or Lazy-S modifications.

Lazy-S

On convex surfaces horizontal contraction will cause a standard fusiform excision to become depressed. The basic fusiform excision may be modified to a Lazy-S shape in these areas. This design increases the total length of the scar so that it is greater than the distance between the two ends. Use of this method allows for contraction along the length of the scar; therefore, the Lazy-S must straighten completely before the scar will become depressed (Figure 4-7).[33,34]

M-Plasty

M-plasty has been used to decrease the overall length of the excision. This modification has to be designed with care to ensure that the midportion of the M does not compromise the recommended surgical margin (Figure 4-8).

Design Problem

Defect Cannot Be Closed

This is probably one of the worst realizations that a surgeon can have. Careful preoperative planning should allow this problem to be avoided. If it does occur, however, consider the following management plan. Do not make things worse by undermining more than 2 cm around the defect or closing the wound under excessive tension. Undermining beyond 2 cm on a fusiform excision yields little additional tissue. The

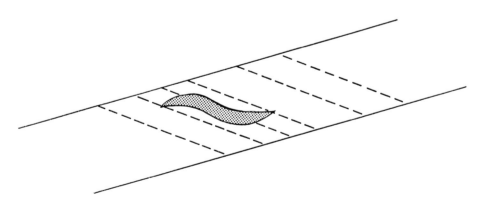

Figure 4.7. Lazy-S design. The central aspect is constructed parallel to the skin tension lines. This design is preferred on convex surfaces.

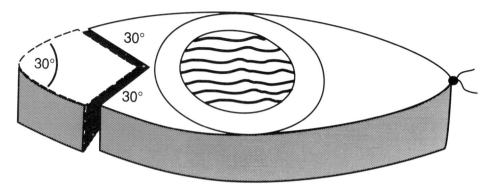

Figure 4.8. M-Plasty. This technique is used to decrease the overall length of the excision while maintaining the preferred 30-degree angles.

temptation to suture the wound closed under undue tension should be resisted, as this may result in wound necrosis, infection, and dehisence. Hemostasis should be ensured and the patient informed that because of the size of the tumor a more complex repair will be needed. In some cases a partial closure may be used to decrease the size of the wound and direct the orientation of the closure. The central aspect of a partial closure can be allowed to heal by second intent or be covered with a full-thickness skin graft. A wound can be left open under a sterile dressing for 5 to 20 days and then repaired without adversely affecting the outcome.[35] An adjacent tissue transfer or skin graft repair should be delayed until the margins are known based on histologic examination. If a delayed closure is to be used, a topical antibiotic ointment should be applied and a sterile dressing placed over the wound. Additionally, oral antibiotic prophylaxis may be recommended.

POSTBIOPSY PLANNING

Histologic Evaluation of an Excisional Biopsy

It is important for the surgeon to know how the patient's tissue is processed. The two most common methods of processing a fusiform shape are breadloaf and breadloaf cross sectioning. In both of these methods a representative sample of the specimen is studied by a pathologist (Figures 4-9 and 4-10). This results in a portion of the tumor and excised surgical margin being examined histologically. These methods have the advantage of lower cost, and they establish the histologic diagnosis along with a sample of excised surgical margin. However, because the entire excised surgical margin is not examined, negative margins are not determined with certainty.

An alternative method of specimen processing is the use of peripheral margins. This method must be requested when the tissue is submitted and is more costly to perform. This approach, however, has the advantage of evaluating the entire excised surgical margin (Figures 4-11 and 4-12). This is especially useful in situations where Mohs

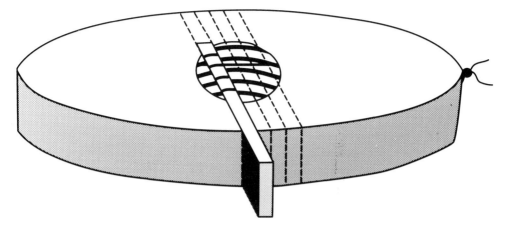

Figure 4.9. Breadloaf sectioning of a fusiform specimen. Each "slice" is examined, resulting in increased sampling of the specimen.

micrographic surgery is not available but where it is important to determine completely that the margins are negative for tumor.[36–40]

Pathology Report

After the biopsy report has been received, the surgeon must determine the requirement for further treatment. The biopsy will have resulted in diagnosis and treatment of most benign cutaneous lesions and in at least the diagnosis of malignant lesions. The biopsy report may not contain, however, adequate information to correctly plan the next surgical step. In the case of basal cell carcinoma and squamous cell carcinoma, it

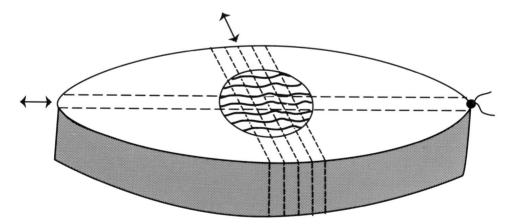

Figure 4.10. Breadloaf–cross sectioning of a fusiform specimen. As in breadloaf sectioning, with the added feature of additional perpendicular sections showing the relationship of the lesion to the tip margins.

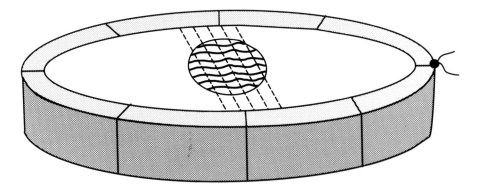

Figure 4.11.   Peripheral margins. This method removes the outer strip of tissue for independent examination, thereby ensuring that the complete lateral margin is examined. The inner portion is then processed in the standard breadloaf style.

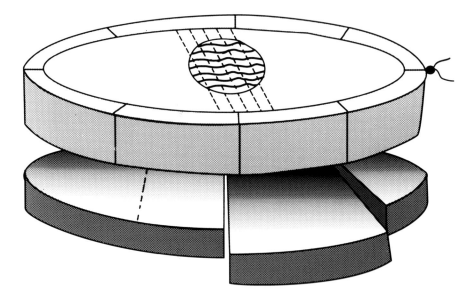

Figure 4.12.   Peripheral margins with separate deep-margin examination. This method is used when the specimen is too thick for a standard tissue cassette. The deep margin of the specimen is separated in the horizontal plane and processed separately. This ensures that all margins have been examined. The remainder of the specimen is processed in the standard breadloaf style.

is not commonplace for the report to contain information such as the depth of tumor invasion using Clark's levels and Breslow measurements. Furthermore, the report may not delineate the tumor subtype. This information might be helpful to the cutaneous surgeon in planning the correct surgical margin and depth of excision for a specific tumor. Examination of the biopsy slide by the surgeon is helpful in supplementing the information contained in the biopsy report. The surgeon is able not only to confirm the pathologic diagnosis but also to gain an appreciation for the extent of the tumor. The purpose of further surgical treatment at this stage is to remove completely any residual tumor with appropriate margins. This final step is best accomplished when the pathology of the lesion is understood.

EXCISIONAL PLANNING FOR REMOVAL OF BASAL AND SQUAMOUS CELL CARCINOMAS

Factors to Consider

Excisional surgery compares favorably to other methods of managing cutaneous malignancies. A multitude of factors must be considered carefully before treating a BCC/SCC malignancy with excisional surgery in order to achieve optimal results. Surgical excision of basal cell carcinoma yields a five-year cure rate of 89.9%.[41] Surgical excision of squamous cell carcinoma yields a five-year cure rate of 91.9%.[42]

Before performing excisional surgery on a cutaneous malignancy, the following factors should be considered: whether the lesion is primary or recurrent, the histology of the lesion, tumor size, anatomic location, perineural spread, and rate of growth. Patient factors such as immunosuppression, previous radiation therapy, carcinogen exposure, lymphoproliferative disorders, organ transplantation, and expectations may also affect the approach. These factors should be used to select the tumors that can be managed using surgical excision without risking a high probability of encountering a positive margin. The initial surgical approach to resect a cutaneous malignant tumor offers the highest cure rate. Recurrent tumors, especially squamous cell carcinomas, have the additional risk of an increased incidence of metastatic spread.

Primary vs Recurrent

Excisional surgery is an excellent treatment modality for primary tumors; however, it is not the treatment of choice for most recurrent tumors. These tumors by their recurrence have demonstrated that their margins were indistinct or that biologically they were more aggressive. In the surgical planning for the removal of recurrent lesions, the clinical margin should include the recurrent tumor and the entire scar from the previous surgery. Around this clinical margin, the surgical margin is drawn.

Recurrence rates for treated BCCs were evaluated by Silverman et al. Although they did not address histologic subtype or amount of surgical margin taken, their data give insight into the expectation of a cure following excisional surgery. The recurrence rate of 588 primary lesions was 4.8%, whereas a recurrence rate of 11.6% occurred in 135 previously treated lesions when excisional surgery was used.[43]

Recurrence rates for treated SCCs were similarly evaluated by Rowe et al. The five-year recurrence rate of 124 primary lesions that were excised was 8.1%; the five-year recurrence rate of 34 locally recurrent lesions that were excised was 23.3%. The danger of metastasis is greatly increased for locally recurrent lesions: 25.1% for skin sites other than ear and lip. The rate was 45% for ear and 31.5% for lip.[42]

Histologic Factors

Subclinical tumor infiltration of 2,016 BCCs has been studied by Breuninger and Dietz. They found that tumors have a highly irregular infiltration pattern with a predilection for small, fingerlike outgrowths when their bases occupied 1–30 degrees of the tumor circumference. Histologic subtype and clinical tumor diameter are the major factors in margin involvement of excisions of basal cell carcinoma, basal cell carcinoma with fibrosis requiring a larger surgical margin.[44]

Squamous cell carcinoma has an incidence of 100,000 cases in the United States each year. These tumors are graded based on their histology from 1 to 4.[45]

Grade 1—More than 75% of cells differentiated
Grade 2—More than 50% of cells differentiated
Grade 3—More than 25% of cells differentiated
Grade 4—Less than 25% of cells differentiated

Grade 1 tumors that do not invade beyond the dermis can be resected using conventional excisional surgery. Histologic features that indicate aggressive behavior are undifferentiated pattern and depth into and beyond the subcutaneous fat. Squamous cell carcinomas carry the additional risk of metastatic disease.

The five-year cure rates of well-differentiated squamous cell carcinoma is 94.6%; for poorly differentiated squamous cell carcinoma it is 61.5%.[42] Tumors that were less than 4 mm in depth/Clark I–III had a local recurrence rate of 5.3% and a metastatic rate of 6.7%. However, tumors greater than 4 mm in depth/Clark IV, V had a local recurrence rate of 17.2% and a metastatic rate of 45.7% (Table 4-2).

Tumor Size

Depending on location and depth, well-defined tumors less than 2 cm in diameter may be managed effectively with conventional excisional surgery. Tumors with diameters greater than 2 cm often demonstrate greater subclinical invasion deep into the subcutaneous fat and may be fixed to underlying structures.

Wolf and Zitelli based their surgical margin recommendations on basal cell carcinomas with well-defined clinical margins less than 2 cm in diameter and found that they could attain clear margins in 95% of cases using a 4-mm surgical margin.[46] Rowe et al evaluated the data on size as a single parameter for behavior of SCC. They found

Table 4.2.   SCC Histology: Recurrence/Metastasis/5 yr-Cure Rate[42]

	Local Recurrence	Metastasis	5-yr Cure
Well differentiated	11.8%	6.0%	94.6%
Poorly differentiated	25.0%	16.4%	61.5%
Neurotropic	47.2%	47.3%	

that tumors less than 2 cm in diameter had a local recurrence rate of 7.4%, and tumors greater than or equal to 2 cm in diameter had a local recurrence rate of 15.2%.[42]

Anatomic Location

Primary basal cell carcinomas located in the following areas have been found to have a high recurrence rate following excisional surgery: ear, 42.9%; nasal-labial groove, 20.2%; scalp, 14.9%; forehead, 8.4%; paranasal, 5.8%; nose, 5.5%; and periocular, 5.3%.[43] Breuninger and Dietz found a higher incidence of fibrosing-type basal cell carcinoma in the H-zone of the face (nose, periocular, and periauricular areas) and felt that the histologic subtype and tumor size alone would predict the need for a larger excisional margin independent of the anatomic site.[35]

Certain anatomic locations are more affected by tumor size. Silverman et al found that increasing tumor size was correlated with higher recurrence rates of basal cell carcinoma of the head but not on the neck, trunk, and extremities, which had a recurrence rate of 0.7% regardless of size.[43] However, in tumors of the head, recurrence rates increased with tumor size: tumors with diameter less than 0.5 cm had a 3.2% recurrence, tumors 0.6 to 0.9 cm had a 8.0% recurrence, and tumors 1 cm or larger had a 9.0% recurrence.

Rowe et al found a high risk for recurrence in squamous cell carcinomas that involved the lip or ear using non-Mohs' modalities followed for five years or more; skin, 7.9%; ear, 18.7%; and lip, 10.5%.[42] Attention must be given to sites of primary squamous cell carcinoma that exhibit a higher degree of metastatic spread: scar carcinoma, 37.9%; lip, 13.7%; and ear, 8.8%.[37]

Perineural Involvement

The presence of perineural spread of a tumor on biopsy necessitates margin control intraoperatively. Perineural tumor spread cannot usually be determined preoperatively. Spread of tumor within the perineural space may go undetected histologically and be left behind following surgery, resulting in recurrence or invasion of critical structures. As a result, conventional excisional surgery has been associated with recurrence rates of 47.2% with squamous cell carcinoma.[42] Squamous cell carcinomas have perineural invasion in 2.4% to 14% of cases; however, basal cell carcinomas have perineural invasion in approximately 1% of cases and must therefore be carefully evaluated histologically as well. Barrett et al believe that these lesions are most effectively managed using Mohs' micrographic surgery, which can trace the involved nerve and continue in a stepwise fashion until the nerve is free of tumor and inflammation. Additionally, they found that the use of postoperative radiation therapy may be beneficial in these patients.[47]

Rapid Growth

Of special concern is a squamous cell carcinoma that has the rapid growth characteristics of a keratoacanthoma. These lesions have a higher metastatic rate: 33% on the ear and eyelid.[48] In our experience, these lesions, although uncommon, are usually treated as keratoacanthomas and then recur. By the time definitive treatment has been obtained, they may have metastasized. Biopsy of all suspected keratoacanthomas is recommended before therapy.

TREATMENT

Effective management of basal cell carcinoma and squamous cell carcinoma using excisional surgery requires that the clinical margin be accurately defined. Even well-defined tumors will have slightly asymmetric growth patterns.[44] The majority of tumors encountered are well-defined primary tumors less than 2 cm in diameter and confined to the dermis, without aggressive histology, rapid growth rate, or perineural involvement. These tumors may be effectively managed using excisional surgery. Additional discretion is required if tumors are located in high-risk areas.

Combined Curettage and Excision Technique

BCCs and SCCs that fit within the parameters described previously may be managed with a slight modification of the combined curettage and excision technique described by Johnson et al.[49] The curette allows for the determination of the inherent asymmetry of even well-defined lesions, enhancing the surgeon's ability to correctly estimate the tumor margin. This technique is not effective in fibrosing tumors or in areas of previous surgery.

The visible margins of the tumor are marked and the lesion is curetted. This curettement should be done aggressively for the deep extent of the tumor and nonaggressively for the peripheral epidermal/dermal margin. The main tumor mass is debulked using a 3- to 6-mm curette, then the subclinical extensions of tumor are delineated using a 2- to 3-mm curette. The clifflike curetted peripheral epidermal margin should be left intact and not be planed by the curette. The resultant defect may have some irregular extensions corresponding to the small, fingerlike outgrowths as described by Breuninger and Dietz.[44]

Spot electrodessication is used to obtain hemostasis. For most tumors the resultant defect will extend 1–2 mm beyond the original clinical margin. This defect reflects the true tumor size and should be measured and recorded as the actual tumor size. Care should be taken using this technique in patients with severe dermatoheliosis. A large area of actinically damaged skin adjacent to the tumor can easily be curetted if the peripheral margin is curetted too aggressively.

After curettement, gentian violet is used to draw around the curetted margin. This is the new clinical margin. Around this margin an appropriate surgical margin is drawn. A fusiform shape is then constructed that is oriented along the relaxed skin tension lines (Figure 4-6). At this time, the proposed excision is evaluated. If the extent of the reconstruction required is beyond the ability of the surgeon, the patient can be referred to a different surgeon at this point.

If it is within the ability of the surgeon to proceed, then one should decide if a primary closure of the fusiform excision is the best or preferred method of reconstruction. If so, then the fusiform is excised as drawn through to the subcutaneous fat. One of the tips is tagged with suture for orientation, and the lesion is separated from the underlying subcutaneous fat.

If the lesion cannot be closed without using an adjacent tissue transfer or full-thickness skin graft, the tumor should be excised as a circle following the surgical margin. The 12-o'clock position of the specimen should be tagged with a suture and a small hash mark placed in the skin using a #15 blade. Closure is delayed until the margins are known histologically.[35]

Surgical Margins for BCC and SCC

A 95% cure rate was obtained for basal cell carcinomas with well-defined clinical margins of 2 cm or less in diameter when a 4-mm margin was used. Basal cell carcinomas do not usually involve the subcutaneous tissue. In the absence of clinical evidence of deep invasion, excision to the midsubcutis is recommended in areas with abundant fatty tissue.[46]

To obtain a 95% cure rate with primary squamous cell carcinomas, a number of factors must be considered. The minimum recommended margin is 4 mm in Grade-1 lesions less than 2 cm in diameter in low-risk areas. Tumors with any one of the following characteristics increase the recommended surgical margin to at least 6 mm: diameter greater than 2 cm, histologic Grade 2 or greater, high-risk location (scalp, ears, eyelids, or nose), and invasion to subcutaneous tissue. Curettement of the lesion may reveal tumor penetration into the subcutaneous fat. Of special concern is that 30% of SCCs extend to the subcutaneous tissue plane. Therefore, it is recommended that all excisions of SCCs include subcutaneous fat. Tumors that have a combination of these factors require 9-mm surgical margins.[50]

Positive Margins

Treatment of a malignancy requires that the lesion be completely excised. If a positive margin is reported, the clinician should examine the histologic slides to gain an appreciation for the extent of tumor involvement. Although SCCs have traditionally been reexcised when a margin was positive, it is now clear that a positive margin following BCC surgery also requires that the lesion be reexcised. This reexcision should be done as soon as the wound has healed.[51] Residual tumor was found at the site of the previous excision in 55% of surgical cases of BCC with positive surgical margins after primary excision when Mohs micrographic surgery was used to remove the residual tumor.[52]

It is less clear how to manage benign tumors that have positive margins on biopsy. It has been our policy to reexcise most of these tumors if they can be excised easily, as benign tumors can also recur and cause local tissue alterations.

SUMMARY

The various techniques discussed in this chapter each have their place in the armamentarium of the dermatologic surgeon. An appropriate biopsy and excisional surgery are the mainstays of diagnosis and management for a variety of benign and malignant lesions. Proper planning and careful patient preparation will result in a well-informed patient with realistic expectations, as well as excellent clinical and histological results.

REFERENCES

1. Zemtsov A, Loring R, Ng TC, et al. Magnetic resonance imaging of cutaneous neoplasms: Clinicopathologic correlation. *J Dermatol Surg Oncol.* 17:416–422, 1991.
2. Zemtsov A. Magnetic resonance imaging in dermatology. *Arch Dermatol.* 129:215–218, 1993.
3. Zemstov A, Reed J, Dixon L. Magnetic resonance imaging evaluation helps to delineate a recurrent skin cancer present under the skin flap. *J Dermatol Surg Oncol.* 18:508–511, 1992.
4. Holzberg M. Glomus tumor of the nail. *Arch Dermatol.* 128:160–162, 1992.
5. Baldwin HE, Berch CM, Lynfield YL. Subcutaneous nodules of the scalp: Preoperative management. *J Am Acad Dermatol.* 25:819–830, 1991.
6. Mohs FE, Snow SN, Kivett WF, Larson PO, Olansky DC, Goldman PM. Anatomic rubber stamps of the face and body to document procedures in dermatologic surgery: One picture is worth a thousand words. *J Dermatol Surg Oncol.* 16:280–291, 1990.
7. Brown CD. Drug interactions in dermatologic surgery. *J Dermatol Surg Oncol.* 18:512–551, 1992.
8. Goldminz D, Bennett RG. Cigarette smoking and flap and full- thickness graft necrosis. *Arch Dermatol.* 127:1012–1015, 1991.
9. Glinert RJ, Zachary CB. Local anesthetic allergy: Its recognition and avoidance. *J Dermatol Surg Oncol.* 17:491–496, 1991.
10. Dajani AS, Bisno AL, Chung KJ, et al. Prevention of bacterial endocarditis: Recommendations by the American Heart Association. *JAMA.* 264:2919–2922, 1990.
11. Nelson JP, Fitzgerald RH, Jaspers MT, Little JW. Prophylactic antimicrobial coverage in arthroplasty patients. *J Bone and Joint Surg.* 72-A:1, 1990.
12. Bencini PL, Galimberti M, Signorini M, Crosti C. Antibiotic prophylaxis of wound infections in skin surgery. *Arch Dermatol.* 127:1357–1360, 1991.
13. Carrick DG. Salicylates and post-tonsillectomy haemorrhage. *J Laryngol and Otol.* 98:803–805, 1984.
14. Nassar RE. The ocular danger of hibiclens (chlorhexidine). *Plast Reconstr Surg.* 89:164–165, 1992.
15. Varley GA, Meisler DM, Benes SC, et al. Hibiclens keratopathy: A clinicopathologic case report. *Cornea.* 9:341–346, 1990.
16. Dresner DL, Lebowitz PW. Atrioventricular sequential pacemaker inhibition by transurethal electrosurgery. *Anesthesiology.* 68:599–601, 1988.
17. Shapiro WA, Roizen MF, Singleton MA, et al. Intraoperative pacemaker complications. *Anesthesiology.* 63:319–322, 1985.
18. Foster CA, Aston SJ. Propranolol-epinephrine interaction: A potential disaster. *Plast Reconstr Surg.* 72:74–78, 1983.
19. Brummett RE. Warning to otolaryngologists using local anesthetics containing epinephrine. *Arch Otolaryngol.* 110:561, 1984.
20. Maloney JM. Local anesthesia obtained via iontophoresis as an aid to shave biopsy. *Arch Dermatol.* 128:331–332, 1992.
21. Stewart JH, Cole GW, Klein JA. Neutralized lidocaine with epinephrine for local anesthesia. *J Dermatol Surg Oncol.* 15:1081–1083, 1989.
22. Larson PO, Ragi G, Swandby M, et al. Stability of buffered lidocaine and epinephrine used for local anesthesia. *J Dermatol Surg Oncol.* 17:411–414, 1991.
23. Pehamberger H, Steiner A, Wolff K. In vivo epiluminescence microscopy of pigmented skin lesions. I. Pattern analysis of pigmented skin lesions. *J Am Acad Dermatol.* 17:571–583, 1987.
24. Kenet RO, Kang S, Kenet BJ, et al. Clinical diagnosis of pigmented lesions using digital epiluminescence microscopy. *Arch Dermatol.* 129:157–174, 1993.
25. Bahmer FA, Fritsch P, Kreusch J, et al. Terminology in surface microscopy. *J Am Acad Dermatol.* 23:1159–1162, 1990.

26. Larson PO. Topical hemostatic agents for dermatologic surgery. *J Dermatol Surg Oncol.* 14:623–632, 1988.
27. Epstein E. Topical hemostatic agents for dermatologic surgery. *J Dermatol Surg Oncol.* 15:342–343, 1989.
28. Rosai J. *Ackerman's Surgical Pathology,* 7th ed. St Louis, MO: CV Mosby; 1989:1932–1934.
29. Gross DA. The vertical wedge biopsy. *J Dermatol Surg Oncol.* 18:630–632, 1992.
30. Grande DJ. Personal communication, 1989.
31. Borges AF. Relaxed skin tension lines. *Dermatol Clinics.* 7:169–177, 1989.
32. Meirson D, Goldberg LH. The influence of age and patient positioning on skin tension lines. *J Dermatol Surg Oncol.* 19:39–43, 1993.
33. Bennett RG. *Fundamentals of Cutaneous Surgery.* St Louis, MO: CV Mosby; 1988:488–489.
34. Zitelli JA. TIPS for a better ellipse. *J Am Acad Dermatol.* 22:101–103, 1990.
35. Mordick T, Hamilton R, Dzubow L. Delayed reconstruction following Mohs surgery for skin cancers of the head and neck. *Am J Surg.* 160:447–449, 1990.
36. Abide JM, Nahai F, Bennett RG. The meaning of surgical margins. *Plast Reconstruc Surg.* 1984;73:492–496.
37. Bennett RG. The meaning and significance of tissue margins. *Adv Dermatol.* 4:343–359, 1989.
38. Freeman RG. Handling of pathologic specimens for gross and microscopic examinations in dermatologic surgery. *J Dermatol Surg Oncol.* 8:673–679, 1982.
39. Hagerty RC, Worshem GF, et al. Peripheral in-continuity tissue examination. *Plast Reconstr Surg.* 83:539–545, 1989.
40. Rapini RP. Comparison of methods for checking surgical margins. *J Am Acad Dermatol.* 23:288–294, 1990.
41. Rowe DE, Carroll RJ, Day CL. Long-term recurrence rates in previously untreated (primary) basal cell carcinoma: Implications for patient follow-up. *J Dermatol Surg Oncol.* 15:315–328, 1989.
42. Rowe DE, Carroll RJ, Day CL. Prognostic factors for local recurrence, metastasis, and survival rates in squamous cell carcinoma of the skin, ear, and lip. *J Am Acad Dermatol.* 26:976–990, 1992.
43. Silverman MK, Kopf AW, Bart RS, et al. Recurrence rates of treated basal cell carcinomas. *J Dermatol Surg Oncol.* 18:471–476, 1992.
44. Breuninger H, Dietz K. Prediction of subclinical tumor infiltration in basal cell carcinoma. *J Dermatol Surg Oncol.* 17:574–578, 1991.
45. Lever WF, Schaumburg-Lever G. *Histopathology of the Skin,* 7th ed. Philadelphia, PA: JB Lippincott; 1990:553–555.
46. Wolf DJ, Zitelli JA. Surgical margins for basal cell carcinoma. *Arch Dermatol.* 123:340–344, 1987.
47. Barrett TL, Greenway HT, Massullo V, et al. Treatment of basal cell carcinoma and squamous cell carcinoma with perineural invasion. *Adv Dermatol.* 8:277–305, 1993.
48. Fitzpatrick PJ, Harwood AA. Acute epithelioma: An aggressive squamous cell carcinoma of the skin. *Am J Clin Oncol.* 8:468–471, 1985.
49. Johnson TM, Tromovitch TA, Swanson NA. Combined curettage and excision: A treatment method for primary basal cell carcinoma. *J Am Acad Dermatol.* 24:613–617, 1991.
50. Brodland DG, Zitelli JA. Surgical margins for excision of primary cutaneous squamous cell carcinoma. *J Am Acad Dermatol.* 27:241–248, 1992.
51. Koplin L, Zarem HA. Recurrent basal cell carcinoma. *Plast Reconstr Surg.* 65:656–664, 1990.
52. Bieley HC, Kirsner RS, Reyes BA, et al. The use of Mohs micrographic surgery for determination of residual tumor in incompletely excised basal cell carcinoma. *J Am Acad Dermatol.* 26:754–756, 1992.

5

SUPERFICIAL ANATOMY OF THE HEAD AND NECK

Eric A. Breisch, PhD

Hubert T. Greenway, MD

INTRODUCTION

Preoperative surgical planning should include a review of the normal anatomic structures in the area where surgery is to be performed. This will allow the dermatologic surgeon to not only provide a better cosmetic result, but also avoid complications related to injury of underlying anatomic structures. Because a significant number of dermatologic surgical procedures are carried out in the head and neck area, the dermatologic surgeon must have a knowledge of the facial nerve and its branches as well as blood vessels, sensory nerves, underlying musculature, and specialized structures such as the parotid duct. This chapter will assist the dermatologic surgeon in his preoperative planning (Figures 5-1 a and b).

BASIC SURFACE ANATOMY OF THE FACE

From the thin and pliable soft tissues of the face the physician can easily identify certain bony prominences and foramina, providing quick reference points for superficial anatomical structures and enabling the clinician to accurately describe and localize regions of the face regarding superficial lesions. With the use of facial diagrams (Figure 5-2) and recorded measurements from these reference points, the exact location of lesions removed can be accurately recorded.

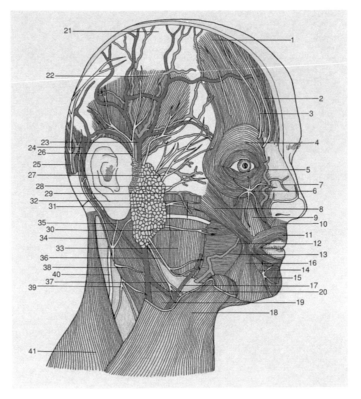

1. Frontalis m.	17. Facial v.	33. Masseter m.
2. Supratrochlear n., a., and v.	18. Platysma m.	34. Lesser occipital n.
3. Supraorbital n.	19. Sternocleidomastoid m.	35. Great auricular n.
4. Orbicularis oculi m.	30. External jugular v.	36. Marginal mandibular branch,
5. Angular a.	21. Galea	facial n.
6. Infraorbital n.	22. Temporalis m.	37. Cervical branch, facial n.
7. Lateral nasal a.	23. Superficial temporal a. and v.	38. Transverse cervical n.
8. Zygomaticus major m.	24. Occipitalis m.	39. Supraclavicular n. (s)
9. Levator labii superioris m.	25. Greater Occipital	40. Spinal accessory n.
10. Depressor septae m.	26. Auriculotemporal n.	41. Trapezius m.
11. Orbicularis oris m.	27. Temporal branch, facial n.	
12. Facial a.	28. Zygomatic branch, facial n.	
13. Buccinator m.	29. Transverse facial artery	
14. Depressor labii inferioris m.	30. Buccal branches, facial n.	
15. Mental n.	31. Parotid gland	
16. Depressor anguli oris m. (triangularis)	32. Parotid duct	

Figure 5.1a.   Superficial Head and Neck Antatomy

The squamous portion of the frontal bone forms the forehead, with laterally positioned rounded projections, called frontal eminences. The bony superciliary arches, located deep behind the eyebrows, are prominent ridges united medially by a small elevation called the glabella. The nasion, a crainometric point located just inferior to the glabella, is formed by the median articulation of the paired nasal bones with the frontal bone. On each side approximately 2 cm lateral from the nasion, along the superior margin of the orbit, is the supraorbital notch, or foramen, which transmits the supraorbital nerve and artery. The supraorbital notch can be palpated in most patients for reference in order to perform a nerve block of the supraorbital nerve. The zygomatic bone forms part of the lateral and inferior margins of the orbit, with the malar portion forming the prominence of the cheek. The temporal process of the zygomatic bone joins the zygo-

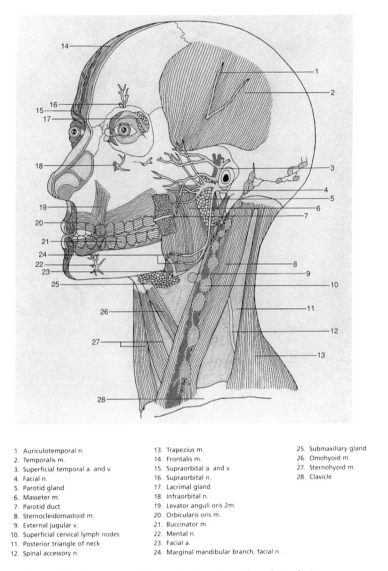

Figure 5.1b.   Superficial and Deep Head and Neck Anatomy

1. Auriculotemporal n.	13. Trapezius m.	25. Submaxillary gland
2. Temporalis m.	14. Frontalis m.	26. Omohyoid m.
3. Superficial temporal a. and v.	15. Supraorbital a. and v.	27. Sternohyoid m.
4. Facial n.	16. Supraorbital n.	28. Clavicle
5. Parotid gland	17. Lacrimal gland	
6. Masseter m.	18. Infraorbital n.	
7. Parotid duct	19. Levator anguli oris 2m.	
8. Sternocleidomastoid m.	20. Orbicularis oris m.	
9. External jugular v.	21. Buccinator m.	
10. Superficial cervical lymph nodes	22. Mental n.	
11. Posterior triangle of neck	23. Facial a.	
12. Spinal accessory n.	24. Marginal mandibular branch, facial n.	

matic process of the temporal bone to form the zygomatic arch. The maxillary bone forms the inferior and medial margins of the orbit, and located in the body of the maxilla, approximately 5 mm below the inferior margin of the orbit, is the infraorbital foramen, which transmits the infraorbital nerve and artery onto the face.

The prominence of the chin is formed by the mental protuberance of the mandible. The body of the mandible lodges the lower dentition and presents a sharp inferior margin. Just lateral to the mental protuberance, the mental foramen is located midway in the height of the body of the mandible.

A vertical line drawn on the face, initiated at the supraorbital foramen and extended inferiorly to the inferior margin of the mandible, will intersect the infraorbital foramen 5 mm below the inferior margin of the orbit and the mental foramen midway

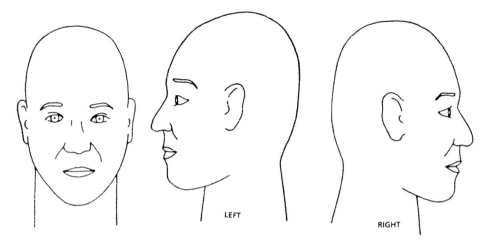

Figure 5.2. Facial diagrams that can be used to record lesion locations. Exact measurements (mm) from anatomic landmarks can be used to further define exact locations.

in the height of the body of the mandible (Figure 5-3). Note that in patients with dentures the position of the mental foramen is best located by measuring approximately 1.0 cm from the inferior margin of the mandible superiorly along the vertical line. This vertical line is a valuable reference line because from it the clinician can quickly identify the surface anatomy of three foramina and their associated sensory nerves.

The body of the mandible ends posteriorly as the angle and the mandible continues superiorly as the ramus. The ramus terminates as the condylar process, which lies directly anterior to the external auditory canal.

The mastoid process of the temporal bone is palpable just behind the auricular cartilage at the level of the external auditory meatus. In the adult the mastoid process protects the main trunk of the facial nerve as it exits the skull through the stylomastoid foramen. The mastoid process is undeveloped at birth and pneumatization of the mastoid region does not begin until approximately five years of age, rendering the facial nerve in this region of the neck at risk during superficial surgical procedures in infants and young children.

FACIAL MUSCULATURE

The muscles of facial expression are all innervated by branches of the facial nerve and in general arise from the facial skeleton to insert into the skin. These muscles are grouped with regard to the region of the face/scalp, ear, periorbital, nose, and mouth where they occur.

Scalp

The most important epicranial muscle of the scalp is the occipitofrontalis muscle (Figure 5-4). The small occipital belly arises from the mastoid process and superior nuchal line of the occipital bone to insert into the galea aponeurosis of the scalp; this muscle pulls the scalp posteriorly. The frontal belly arises from the anterior aspect of

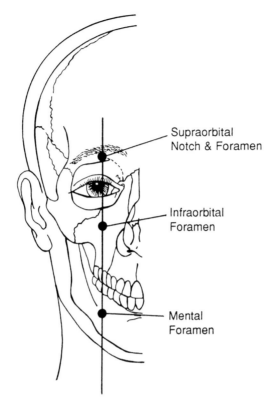

Supraorbital
Notch & Foramen

Infraorbital
Foramen

Mental
Foramen

Figure 5.3.   Supraorbital notch (palpable) above the eye is in direct alignment with the infraorbital and mental foramen. Normally these are *not* in the midpupilary line.

the galea aponeurosis and inserts into the skin of the forehead and eyebrows; it acts to pull the scalp anteriorly and elevates the eyebrows. The occipital belly is innervated by the posterior auricular branch of the facial nerve, and the frontal belly is innervated by the temporal branch of the facial nerve.

Ear

The anterior auricular muscle, superior auricular muscle, and posterior auricular muscle arise from the scalp and insert into the skin and auricle as their names suggest (Figure 5-4). Functionally, these muscles are of no clinical importance and are innervated by posterior and temporal branches of the facial nerve. However, these muscles are highly vascularized and may be incorporated as musculo-cutaneous flaps in staged pedicle ear reconstructions.

Periorbital

The muscles of the eyelid include the orbicularis oculi, levator palpebrae superioris, corrugator supercilii, and procerus (Figure 5-5). The orbicularis oculi muscle is a concentrically arranged muscle that is typically divided into two parts: palpebral and orbital. The palpebral part is that portion of the muscle which covers the eyelid; it orig-

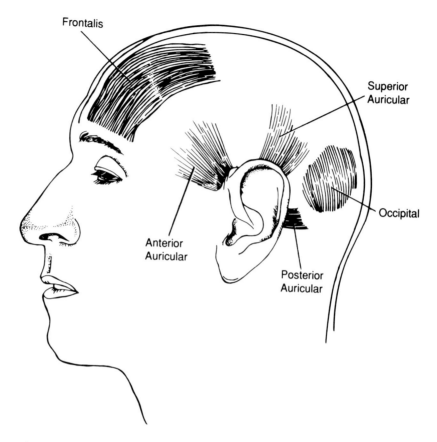

Figure 5.4.   Scalp and ear musculature. Auricular muscles may vary considerably in development.

inates from the superior and inferior aspect of the medial palpebral ligament. Fibers pass laterally in both the upper and lower lids to interdigitate finally at the lateral aspect of the eyelid, thereby forming the lateral palpebral raphe. The orbital part of the orbicularis oculi muscle originates from the medial palpebral ligament, the frontal process of the maxillary bone, and the nasal process of the frontal bone; its fibers extend out beyond the bony margins of the orbit in a series of concentric loops to insert into the overlying skin in the regions of the forehead, as well as the malar and infraorbital areas of the cheek. The palpebral part of this muscle acts to close the eyelid gently, while the orbital part is used for blinking and tight closure of the eyelid. The motor innervation of the orbicularis oculi muscle is from the temporal and zygomatic branches of the facial nerve. Paralysis of these nerve branches leads to ectropion of the lid and inability to close the lids. Even temporary paralysis from a local anesthetic may require temporary patching of the eye to protect the cornea.

The levator palpebrae superioris muscle originates from the apex of the orbit and extends forward, forming a broad aponeurosis that inserts into the superior aspect of the superior tarsal plate. Its action is to elevate the upper eyelid, thereby widening the

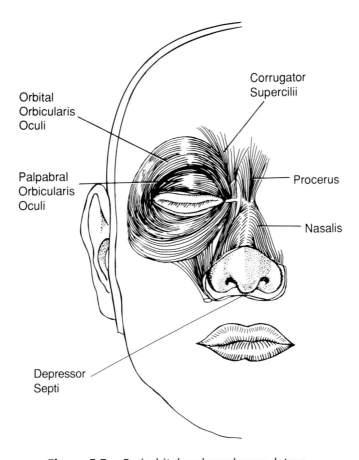

Figure 5.5. Periorbital and nasal musculature.

palpebral fissure. This muscle is innervated by the superior division of the oculomotor nerve; paralysis leads to ptosis of the lid.

The corrugator supercilii muscle arises from the medial part of the superciliary ridge to insert into the skin of the eyebrow; it pulls the eyebrows medially. This muscle is innervated by the temporal branches of the facial nerve.

The procerus muscle originates from the superior aspect of the nasal bones to insert into the skin overlying the root of the nose; it pulls the medial aspect of the eyebrows inferiorly. The procerus muscle is innervated by the temporal branches of the facial nerve.

Nose

The muscles of the nose are highly variable in their development and consist of the nasalis (Figure 5-4) and depressor septi muscles.

The transverse portion of the nasalis muscle originates from the body of the maxilla and, along with its associate from the opposite side, inserts into an aponeurotic sling that passes over the bridge of the nose. A smaller, alar portion of this muscle inserts into the lateral crus of the alar cartilage of the nose. The transverse portion of the nasalis compresses the nares, while the alar portion dilates the nares. In the removal of cutaneous malignancies that invade deeply and invade the nasalis, removal may cause the loss of this function; even a precise nasal reconstruction may not completely restore this compression/dilation activity. The nasalis muscle is innervated by the buccal branches of the facial nerve.

The depressor septi muscle, arising from the incisive fossa of the maxilla, inserts into the columella and nasal septum; it narrows the nares. This muscle is innervated by the buccal branches of the facial nerve.

Mouth

The muscles associated with the mouth arise from different regions on the face to insert into the skin and mucosa of the mouth. Initially this seems like a complex area to learn because of the large number of muscles. Clinically, one may wish to divide them into the depressor group of the lower lip, the elevator group of the upper lip, the buccinator cheek wall muscle, and the orbicularis muscle of the lip proper.

The muscles of the lower lip are the depressor anguli oris, the depressor labii inferioris, the mentalis, and the platysma (Figure 5-6).

The depressor anguli oris muscle arises from the anterolateral aspect of the body of the mandible, inserts into the skin and mucosa at the labial commissure, and depresses the corner of the mouth.

The depressor labii inferioris muscle originates from the mandible just deep to the depressor anguli oris muscle; it inserts into the skin and mucosa of the lower lip and depresses the lower lip.

The mentalis muscle, arising from the body of the mandible medial to the depressor labii inferioris muscle, inserts into the skin overlying the tip of the chin, effecting protrusion of the lower lip and dimpling of the skin.

The platysma muscle is a superficial muscle of the neck; its fibers ascend from the neck onto the face to insert into the skin of the lower lip and labial commissure. This muscle helps to depress the lower lip and pull the angle of the mouth inferolaterally.

All the lower lip muscles except the platysma are innervated by the marginal mandibular branch of the facial nerve, with secondary innervation from the buccal branches of the facial nerve; the platysma muscle is innervated by the cervical branches of the facial nerve.

The musculature of the upper lip consists of the risorius, zygomaticus major and minor, levator labii superioris, levator labii superioris alaeque nasi, and levator anguli oris muscles.

The risorius muscle originates from the parotid fascia, passes anteriorly to insert into the skin and mucosa at the corner of the mouth, and pulls the labial commissure laterally, widening the mouth.

The zygomaticus major muscle, originating from the posterolateral aspect of the zygomatic bone, inserts into the skin and mucosa of the lateral upper lip and elevates the labial commissure.

The zygomaticus minor muscle, arising just medial to the zygomaticus major muscle, inserts into the skin and mucosa of the upper lip and elevates the upper lip.

The levator labii superioris muscle arises from the maxilla just above the infraor-

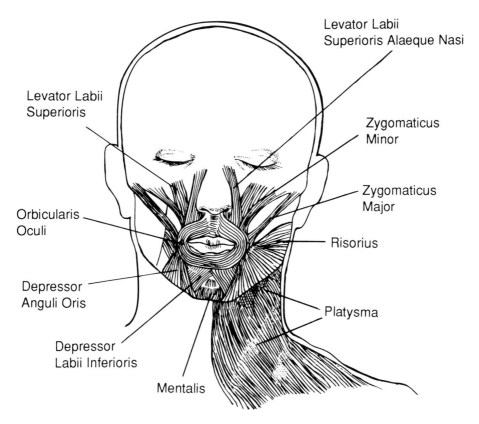

Levator Labii
Superioris Alaeque Nasi

Levator Labii
Superioris

Zygomaticus
Minor

Zygomaticus
Major

Orbicularis
Oculi

Risorius

Depressor
Anguli Oris

Platysma

Depressor
Labii Inferioris

Mentalis

Figure 5.6.   Muscles of the mouth region.

bital foramen and inserts into the skin and mucosa of the medial upper lip; it is an elevator of the upper lip.

The levator labii superioris alaeque nasi muscle, arising from the medial margin of the orbit, first passes fibers into the ala of the nose, continues inferiorly, and finally inserts into the medial aspect of the skin and mucosa of the upper lip. This muscle is an elevator of the lip and dilates the nares.

The levator anguli oris muscle originates from the maxilla just below the infraorbital foramen and inserts into the skin and mucosa at the labial commissure; this muscle elevates the corner of the mouth.

The muscles associated with the upper lip are innervated by the buccal branches of the facial nerve, with secondary innervation from the zygomatic branches of the facial nerve.

The buccinator muscle forms the muscular wall of the cheek, arising from the posterolateral aspect of the maxilla, the medial aspect of the mandible near the last molar, and the pterygomandibular raphe; it inserts into the skin and mucosa of the labial commissure and the upper and lower lips. This muscle flattens the lips and cheeks against the teeth. The buccinator is innervated by the buccal branches of the facial nerve and is the only muscle of facial expression to receive its innervation from the superficial aspect.

The orbicularis oris muscle is the chief muscle of the lips and consists of concentrically arranged fibers that circumscribe the mouth and insert into the skin and mucosa surrounding the mouth. These fibers provide a sphincteral function, allowing pursing and protrusion of the lips. The orbicularis oris muscle is innervated by the buccal branches of the facial nerve. In lip reconstruction such as after a lip wedge excision, the orbicularis oris muscle must be reconstructed as a separate muscle layer to restore its sphincteric function. Topographically before lip surgery, the surgeon may wish to mark the vermilion border (with an inked pen or temporary sutures) so as to recreate it exactly after the underlying muscle repair. Finally, the reconstruction of the lateral commissure may require special attention due to the action of the surrounding muscles that insert into that area.

THE SUPERFICIAL MUSCULAR APONEUROTIC SYSTEM (SMAS)

SMAS consists of muscle and a thin layer of superficial fascia that invests all the muscles of facial expression. This fascial layer envelops the facial muscles more distinctly and definitively in certain areas, specifically the lower face, midface, and forehead regions. The fascial component of SMAS originates as the superficial cervical fascial layer, envelops the platysma muscle, sweeps over the mandible, and invests the muscles of the face. The superficial fascia is tightly adherent to the mastoid process of the temporal bone, the deep fascia investing the sternocleidomastoid muscle, the fascia of the parotid gland approximately 1–2 cm anterior to the tragus, with points of attachment to the periosteum of the zygomatic arch via fine fascicula. The fascia is very thin within the temporal zone and is difficult to separate from the deep temporal fascia.

Functionally, the fascia provides a network that binds together nearly all the muscles of facial expression, allowing them to act in concert with one another, providing a method for evenly distributing the pull of the muscles on the overlying skin, and acting as a fire wall to prevent the spread of infection from superficial to deep areas of the face.

THE PRIMARY RESTING SKIN TENSION LINES

The muscles of facial expression have their insertion into the overlying skin, and the resulting pull causes the skin to fold or crease in regular pattern. These creases are referred to as resting skin tension lines (RSTL); typically they occur perpendicular to the long axis of the underlying muscle (Figure 5-7). Incisions made parallel to these lines produce a fine, linear scar while incisions made perpendicular to these lines may produce an irregular, hypertrophic scar. The position of RSTL on the face is usually very predictable, although certain areas of the face seem to contradict the prediction formula for RSTL, eg, the periorbital region. However, because SMAS is very tenuous in the periorbital region, the muscle attachment to the overlying skin is very weak, thereby permitting RSTL to be primarily influenced by gravity and muscles of the orbit. To best demonstrate the position of the RSTL, ask the patient to perform a variety of exaggerated facial expressions, which should help predict the position of the RSTL.

The RSTL of the forehead are oriented horizontally because of the frontalis muscle. In the region of the glabella RSTL can be found as vertical lines owing to the cor-

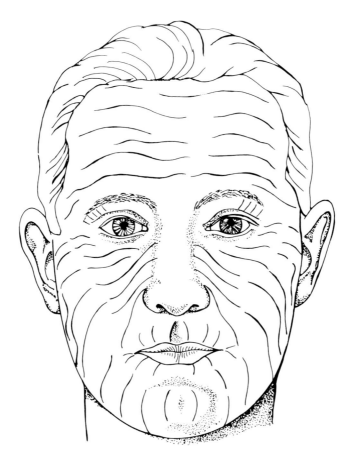

Figure 5.7. The primary resting skin tension lines. Note these normally occur perpendicular to the long axis of the underlying muscle.

rugator supercilii muscle and transverse lines over the nasion owing to the pull of the procerus muscle.

The periorbital regions demonstrate radial lines at the medial and lateral canthus owing to the orbicularis oculi muscle. The RSTL of the lids are horizontal owing to the pull of gravity and the levator palpebrae superioris muscle of the orbit.

The skin of the nose demonstrates no predictable RSTL. The skin of the midface and perioral region demonstrate the expected RSTL. The pull of the orbicularis oris causes skin tension lines to radiate from the perimeter of the mouth. The zygomaticus muscles help accentuate the melolabial fold, while the risorius muscle helps create the vertical skin folds found over the cheek.

It should be remembered that some variation of the RSTL will occur from one individual to the next. Secondary skin tension lines, which frequently occur perpendicular to RSTL, can result from aging of the skin, sun damage, altered states of hydration, or redundant folds of skin owing to recent weight loss. Normally the best cosmetic results may be obtained by planning excisions with subsequent closures within or parallel to skin tension lines. At times the surgeon may violate this principle to protect a critical underlying structure such as a superficial branch of the facial nerve.

BLOOD SUPPLY OF THE FACE

The arterial supply to the face is a network derived from branches of the external carotid and the internal carotid arteries (Figure 5-8).

The facial artery is a branch of the external carotid artery in the neck; it ascends along the lateral aspect of the pharynx, grooves the submandibular gland, then hooks upward around the mandible to reach the face. It is easily palpated as it crosses the mandible at the anterior edge of the insertion of the masseter muscle and passing superficial to the buccinator muscle, the artery pursues a tortuous course toward the medial angle of the eye. The first branches arising from the facial artery are the inferior and superior labial arteries, which anastomose freely with their associates from the opposite side and weave sinuously through the muscle fibers of the orbicularis oris muscle. The facial artery continues as the angular artery and as it runs along the lateral margin of the nose toward the eye it supplies the lateral nasal artery, which supplies most of the external nose.

The inferior labial artery reinforces the mental artery from the inferior alveolar artery over the chin. The facial artery has many small muscular branches that anastomose freely in the cheek with the buccal artery, derived from the maxillary artery; the infraorbital artery, derived from the maxillary artery; and the transverse facial artery, derived from the superficial temporal artery.

The facial artery terminates at the medial aspect of the eye as the angular artery, freely communicating with the supraorbital artery, supratrochlear artery, and dorsal nasal artery, all derived from the ophthalmic artery via the internal carotid artery.

The temporal region is supplied by the superficial temporal artery, the terminal branch of the external carotid artery. The forehead receives the frontal branch of the superficial temporal artery and is reinforced by the supraorbital and supratrochlear arteries. The posterior scalp is supplied by the occipital and postauricular arteries, derived from the external carotid artery. The remainder of the scalp is supplied via branches from the occipital, postauricular, superficial temporal, and supraorbital arteries.

In practice, the most common arteries requiring suture ligation are the superficial temporal artery and its branches, and the labial artery systems. While an electric cautery can seal a number of small vessels, it is important to remember that the arterial system circulates at high pressure. The epinephrine in local anesthetics may cause initial vasoconstriction with delayed postoperative bleeding after this effect has worn off where vessels were not sufficiently handled. In our practice we find that episodes of delayed bleeding most commonly occur in the ear.

The venous system of the face parallels the arterial distribution. The lateral forehead region drains into the superficial temporal vein. The medial forehead drains into the supratrochlear and supraorbital veins, which communicate with the ophthalmic venous system, and the angular vein at the medial aspect of the eye. The angular vein descends along the lateral aspect of the nose and receives the venous drainage of the nose. The angular vein is joined by the superior and inferior labial veins to form the anterior facial vein. The anterior facial vein crosses the inferior margin of the mandible just posterior to the facial artery and finally drains into the internal jugular vein. The temporal and parietal scalp, anterolateral ear, and posterior facial regions drain into the superficial temporal vein, which joins the maxillary vein to form the retromandibular vein. The retromandibular vein passes through the parotid gland and bifurcates into an anterior and a posterior branch. The anterior branch

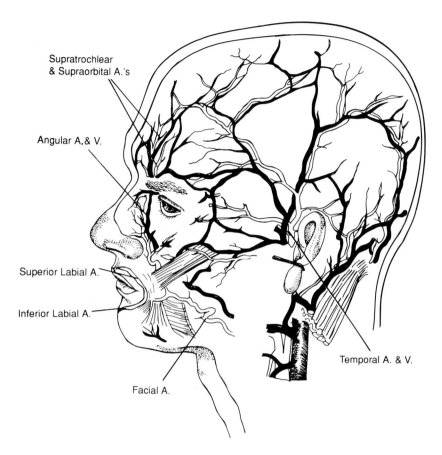

Supratrochlear
& Supraorbital A.'s

Angular A.& V.

Superior Labial A.

Inferior Labial A.

Temporal A. & V.

Facial A.

Figure 5.8.   Blood supply of the face and scalp. While mainly external carotid branches, a number of other branches are derived from the internal carotid artery. The venous system parallels the arterial distribution.

joins the anterior facial vein, and the posterior division joins the posterior auricular vein to form the external jugular vein.

LYMPHATICS OF THE HEAD

The lymphatic system of the scalp and face drains into regionally located lymph nodes found in close association with the primary venous pathways (Figure 5-9).

The occipital region drains into scattered occipital nodes found along the superior nuchal lines. The retroauricular nodes, located over the mastoid process, receive lymphatic drainage from the occipital, parietal, and temporal scalp as well as the postero-medial auricle.

The forehead, temporal, and lateral canthal regions drain into preauricular or superficial parotid nodes. The medial eyelids, nose, cheek, and upper lip drain into the scattered facial nodes that parallel the facial vein.

The lips and mental region drain into submental and submandibular nodes located within the neck. The upper lips (right and left) drain into the ipsilateral submandibular nodes; the lateral aspect of the lower lips drain into the ipsilateral submandibular nodes, and the medial aspect of the lower lips drain into ipsilateral and contralateral submental and submandibular lymph nodes.

In lesions with metastatic potential it is important to examine (and document in the medical record) the anatomic areas of most likely lymphatic drainage preoperatively to assess the status for metastatic spread. The presence of lymphadenopathy in such a case requires further evaluation. Further radiologic tests (CT, MRI) can be helpful in assessing the condition of the lymphatic nodes. Fine needle aspiration (FNA) of an enlarged palpable node may be indicated.

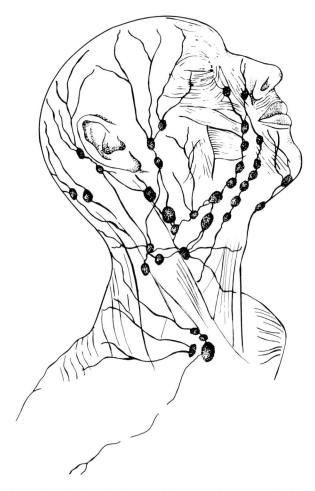

Figure 5.9.   Lymphatic drainage of the head and neck. Assessment of anatomic areas of likely drainage is indicated in those lesions with metastatic potential.

THE PAROTID GLAND

The parotid gland, positioned superficial to the masseter muscle, is not palpable, lies on the side of the face just anterior to the ear, and has a somewhat triangular configuration (Figures 5-10, 5-11). The superior pole of the parotid gland is located just anterior to the ear and immediately below the zygomatic arch; the inferior pole extends below to nearly the angle of the mandible. The gland's posterior margin parallels the posterior edge of the ramus of the mandible, and its isthmus lies wedged between the external auditory canal and the ramus of the mandible; the anterior border lies superficial to the masseter muscle, extending a variable distance anteriorly. The parotid duct emerges from the anterior border of the gland, crosses the masseter, then penetrates the buccinator muscle to empty into the buccal vestibule opposite the second upper molar. The duct is easily palpable at the anterior edge of the masseter at a point midway between the zygomatic arch and the labial commissure. The parotid gland provides protection for the facial nerve and its main branches. Normally it is not encountered or violated during removal of overlying cutaneous tumors except in recurrent or special cases. However, if one encounters a tumor invading the underlying parotid, consideration must be given for a parotidectomy.

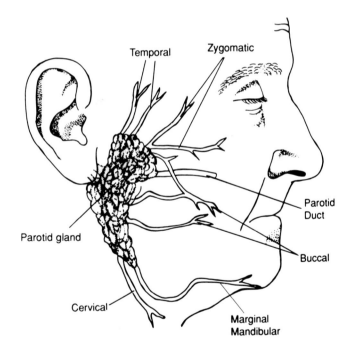

Figure 5.10.   Branches of the facial nerve.
Temporal
Zygomatic
Buccal
Marginal Mandibular
Cervical

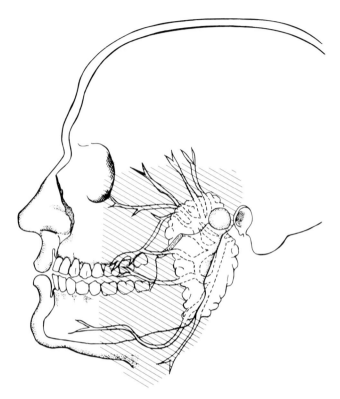

Figure 5.11.   The danger zone (shaded area) of the facial nerve where because of the anatomy branches may be more at risk for injury (see text).

THE FACIAL NERVE

The main stem of the facial nerve emerges through the base of the skull via the stylomastoid foramen. The first extracranial branch, the posterior auricular, passes posteriorly to supply the occipital belly of the occipitofrontalis muscle and the posterior auricular muscle. The facial nerve continues anteriorly through the neck to penetrate the deep surface of the parotid gland, which protects the nerve during its intraparotid course. Within the parotid gland the facial nerve divides into five major branches (temporal, zygomatic, buccal, marginal mandibular, and cervical), which then leave the parotid gland (Figure 5-10) and are named for the region of the face they supply (Table 5-1).

The extraparotid course of the facial nerve branches may be divided into safe and danger zones. The danger zone (Figure 5-11) is delineated by a line drawn 1 cm above and parallel to the zygomatic arch, starting at the auricle and finishing at the lateral margin of the orbit. Then a vertical line is drawn from the lateral margin of the orbit inferiorly to the inferior margin of the mandible at the insertion of the masseter muscle; this is connected to a line curving 2 cm below the mandible to terminate at the angle of the mandible posteriorly. The area circumscribed by these boundaries on the posterior face is defined as the danger zone of the facial nerve. The branches of the facial nerve have not arborized extensively within this danger zone; cutting a nerve branch in this area may cause a motor deficit. Even local anesthesia within the danger zone (somewhat in the shape of a letter "C," around the anterior border of the parotid) may cause temporary motor deficit. The area outside the danger zone is called the safe zone, because the facial nerve branches have extensively arborized; injuring a small peripheral branch in this zone creates no significant motor deficits except for possibly the marginal mandibular branch.

The temporal branches of the facial nerve leave the superior pole of the parotid gland, pass superficial to the zygomatic arch to supply the anterior and superior auricular muscles, the orbicularis oculi muscle, the frontal belly of the occipitofrontalis muscle, the corrugator supercilii muscle, and the procerus muscle. Damage to the nerve may cause drooping of the ipsilateral eyelid and inability to close the lid tightly. Clinically, the temporal branch is the most commonly injured one, probably because of its superficial location and the large number of tumors occurring in that area. It may be acceptable and even required to remove a portion of the nerve for a deeply invading tumor; however, it is not acceptable to violate an intact nerve during reconstructive or cosmetic procedures. The drooping of the eyelid related to lack of innervation of the frontalis muscle can be significantly problematic to the patient. Surgical repair procedures may include a forehead lift, a brow lift, and a blepharoplasty on the affected side. For nonsurgical repairs (such as in cases of anesthesia), surgical tape may be used temporarily to elevate the sagging brow.

The zygomatic branches of the facial nerve leave the anterosuperior aspect of the parotid gland and proceed toward the lateral angle of the eye. These branches supply the orbicularis oculi muscle and the zygomaticus major and minor muscles, with secondary innervation to the levators of the lip. Damage to this branch results in an ectropion of the lower eyelid, weakness in blinking, tight closure of the eyelid, and moderate facial asymmetry when smiling. Patching of the eye may be required to protect the cornea.

The buccal branches emerge from the anterior border of the parotid gland and parallel the parotid duct, supplying the buccinator muscle, risorius muscle, orbicularis oris muscle, levators of the lip, depressor septi muscle, and nasalis muscle, with secondary innervation to the depressor anguli and depressor labii inferioris muscles. Injury to these branches results in weakness in the oral sphincter (unable to whistle or pucker lips).

The marginal mandibular branches of the facial nerve exit the inferior pole of the parotid gland to parallel the inferior margin of the mandible. In elderly patients these

Table 5.1. Facial Nerve

Branch	Muscle Innervation*	Deficit
Temporal	Frontalis	Brow sag, to Ptosis
Zygomatic	Orb. Oculi	Inability to close eye tightly
Buccal	Lip elevators	Unopposed pull normal side
M. mandibular	Lip depressors	Unopposed pull normal side
Cervical	Platysma	Minimal in man

*Crossover may exist

nerve branches may descend 2 cm below the inferior margin of the mandible before they ascend back up into the face at the insertion site of the masseter muscle onto the mandible. The marginal mandibular branches continue forward, superficial to the facial artery and vein, to innervate the depressor anguli oris, depressor labii inferioris, and mentalis muscles. Damage to these branches causes facial asymmetry when talking or smiling. Injury to the buccal branches or the marginal mandibular branches (thus the elevators and depressors of the lips) may clinically result in asymmetry from unopposed pull from the normal side.

The cervical branches of the facial nerve emerge from the inferior pole of the parotid gland, descend behind the angle of the mandible into the neck, and innervate the platysma muscle. Clinically, the loss of platysma function on one side in the human face may not be overly self-evident.

Most commonly, facial nerve damage and deficits are temporary, relating to local anesthesia in cutaneous surgical procedures. The tincture of time (relating to short- versus long-acting local anesthesia) is the cure with patient management (ie, an eye patch) as required. However, if one does inadvertently cut a branch of the facial nerve, immediate repair is indicated and can be successfully completed but requires special techniques and assistance.

SENSORY INNERVATION OF THE FACE AND SCALP

The skin of the face receives its principal sensory innervation from the trigeminal nerve. The three divisions of the trigeminal nerve—ophthalmic, maxillary, and mandibular—designate the area of the face they supply.

Ophthalmic Division

The supraorbital and supratrochlear nerves supply skin over the medial upper eyelid, forehead, and scalp as far superiorly as the crown.

The infratrochlear nerve innervates skin over the medial upper eyelid and bridge of the nose.

The lacrimal nerve supplies skin over the lateral upper eyelid.

The dorsal external nasal nerve is the terminal branch of the anterior ethmoidal nerve and supplies a strip of skin over the dorsum of the nose down to the tip.

Maxillary Division

The infraorbital nerve supplies the skin of the lower eyelids, lateral sides of the nose, upper lips, and buccal cheek.

The zygomatic nerve splits into the zygomaticofacial and zygomaticotemporal nerves, which supply skin over the malar region of the cheek and anterior temporal scalp region.

Mandibular Division

The mental nerve innervates the skin of the chin and lower lip, extending laterally to the labial commissure.

The buccal nerve descends into the cheek, between the temporalis and buccinator muscles, to supply the skin of the buccal cheek.

The auriculotemporal nerve, accompanying the superficial temporal artery, supplies the upper anterolateral quadrant of the auricle, anterior half of the external auditory canal and tympanic membrane, and most of the temporal scalp region.

The use of nerve blocks of the various divisions of the trigeminal nerve may be advantageous in certain situations to provide better local anesthesia. Chapter 6 pages 102–107 further delineates sensory innervation and the use of various nerve blocks (i.e. supraorbital, infraorbital, mental).

BASIC TOPOGRAPHY ANATOMY OF THE NECK

Several bony and cartilaginous structures are palpable in the neck and serve as useful reference points.

Approximately two finger breadths below the chin, the body of the hyoid bone is identified in midline. Below the hyoid bone the prominence of the thyroid cartilage is palpated in midline. The anterior lamina of the cricoid cartilage is situated just below the thyroid cartilage. The small gap between the thyroid and cricoid is filled by the cricothyroid ligament and represents an important site for emergency access to the airway. Inferior to the cricoid are the prominent tracheal rings.

Posteriorly, the external occipital protuberance, palpable in midline over the occipital bone, marks the superiormost reference point of the posterior neck. With the neck flexed, the first palpable spinous process is that of the seventh cervical vertebra (vertebra prominens), demarcating the base of the neck.

Clinically, the vertebra prominens is an important topical landmark. One can document lesions laterally by measuring the number of centimeters from this point.

Triangles of the Neck

The boundaries of the anterior triangle of the neck are as follows: the mastoid process of the temporal bone, the tip of the chin, the midpoint of the jugular notch, and the anterior border of the sternocleidomastoid muscle (Figure 5-12). This triangle can be subdivided into four smaller triangles: the submandibular, the submental, the carotid, and the muscular. The submandibular triangle, delineated by lines drawn from the mastoid process to the tip of the chin, to the lesser cornu of the hyoid bone and back to the mastoid process, contains the submandibular gland, facial artery and vein, branches of the facial nerve (cervical and marginal mandibular), and lymph nodes. The carotid triangle, bounded by lines drawn from the mastoid process to the lesser cornu of the hyoid, from the hyoid to the junction of the lower third with the middle third of the anterior border of the sternocleidomastoid muscle and back to the mastoid process, contains the carotid arteries, internal jugular vein, and associated lymph nodes. The submental triangle contains scattered lymph nodes and is bounded by a line drawn from the tip of the chin to the middle of the hyoid bone, laterally to the lesser cornu of the hyoid, and back to the tip of the chin. The muscular triangle, extending from the middle of the hyoid, inferiorly to the manubrium, along the anterior edge of the sternocleidomastoid muscle to its junction of the lower third with the middle third, back to the middle of the hyoid, contains the thyroid gland.

The posterior cervical triangle (Figure 5-12), the apex of which initiates at the mastoid process, is bounded posteriorly by the anterior edge of the trapezius muscle and anteriorly by the posterior border of the sternocleidomastoid muscle, and inferiorly along the base by the clavicle. The most important superficial structure located within the posterior cervical triangle is the spinal accessory nerve, which emerges from the posterior border of the sternocleidomastoid muscle and crosses the triangle obliquely to penetrate the anterior edge of the trapezius muscle. The spinal accessory nerve is at risk during its entire course through the posterior cervical triangle, because it is covered only by the superficial cervical fascia and skin. Note that the platysmal muscle does *not* cover the spinal accessory nerve in the posterior cervical triangle. The nerve innervates the trapezius muscle, and resultant damage to the nerve during its superficial course may result in an inability to elevate the shoulder on the affected side. Thus, in procedures in this area one may wish to have the patient elevate his or her shoulder periodically to ensure continued function. The external jugular vein, formed near the angle of the mandible, descends vertically across the sternocleidomastoid muscle, finally emptying into the subclavian vein at the base of the posterior cervical triangle.

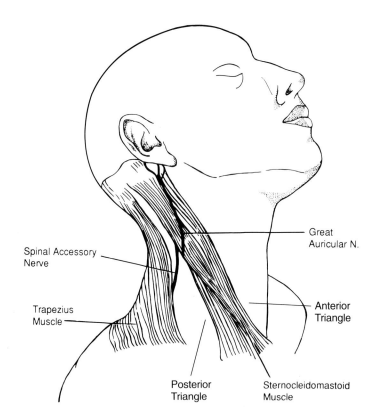

Figure 5.12. Important anatomic structures of the neck of concern in dermatologic surgical procedures. Note that the spinal accessory nerve is not protected by the platysma muscle in the posterior triangle of the neck.

SUPERFICIAL CERVICAL MUSCULATURE

The platysma muscle, covering nearly the entire anterior triangle of the neck from the clavicle to the mandible, arises from the upper thoracic fascia to insert into the skin of the lower face and lower lateral lip. The platysma muscle, tensing the skin over the neck and pulling the lower lip inferiorly and laterally, is innervated by the cervical branches of the facial nerve. This muscle never overlies the accessory spinal nerve within the posterior cervical triangle and covers only the most inferior aspect of the posterior cervical triangle. The sternocleidomastoid muscle, extending obliquely across the neck, originates from the clavicle and sternum, inserts into the mastoid process of the temporal bone, and is innervated by the spinal accessory nerve.

BLOOD SUPPLY OF THE NECK

The arterial supply to the overlying skin and superficial structures located within the posterior and anterior cervical triangles is derived via penetrating branches from the deeply positioned external carotid artery and thyrocervical trunk.

The superficial veins of the neck consist of the anterior and external jugular venous systems. The anterior jugular vein, located just deep to the platysma muscle, originates within the submental triangle, descends toward the lower aspect of the muscular triangle, and passes posterior to the sternocleidomastoid muscle to terminate in the external jugular vein. The external jugular vein is formed over the sternocleidomastoid muscle by the union of the postauricular vein with the posterior division of the retromandibular vein; it descends vertically to enter the subclavian vein within the posterior cervical triangle.

The lymphatics of the superficial structures of the neck drain into the nodes of the superficial cervical lymphatic chain, which parallels the external jugular vein. The scattered nodes found in the submental and submandibular triangles drain into the jugulodigastric node, with direct drainage into the deep cervical lymphatic chain.

Just as with the facial lymphatics, the lymphatics of the neck must be evaluated and recorded where there exists a possibility of metastatic spread.

MOTOR AND SENSORY NERVES OF THE NECK

The main stem of the facial nerve emerges from the base of the skull through the stylomastoid foramen and quickly penetrates the posterior aspect of the parotid gland. Within the parotid gland the facial nerve splits into five terminal branches (temporal, zygomatic, buccal, marginal mandibular, and cervical). Only the cervical and marginal mandibular branches have important relationships in the neck. The cervical branches of the facial nerve exit from the inferior pole of the parotid gland and descend below the angle of the mandible to innervate the platysma muscle. The marginal mandibular branch of the facial nerve normally parallels the inferior margin of the mandible, but in the elderly frequently descends into the submandibular triangle of the neck before it ascends back up into the face to supply the lower lip musculature.

The spinal accessory nerve emerges from approximately the junction of the upper third and middle third of the posterior border of the sternocleidomastoid muscle, passes inferiorly and obliquely across the posterior cervical triangle, and innervates the trapezius muscle. The spinal accessory nerve is at risk during its entire passage within the posterior cervical triangle because it is covered only by thin skin and a layer of fascia.

The cutaneous innervation of the neck is provided via branches from the cervical plexus. These nerves emerge from the posterior edge of the sternocleidomastoid muscle at approximately its midpoint to supply the overlying skin of the anterior and posterior cervical triangles. The lesser occipital nerve ascends along the posterior border of the sternocleidomastoid muscle, supplying skin overlying the apex of the posterior cervical triangle, posteromedial auricle, and occipital scalp. The greater auricular nerve crosses superficial to the sternocleidomastoid muscle, ascends directly toward the auricle, and supplies the skin overlying the upper half of the sternocleidomastoid muscle, posteromedial and anterolateral auricles, and posterior and inferior regions of the face. The transverse cervical nerves cross the superficial aspect of the sternocleidomastoid muscle horizontally, supplying skin overlying the anterior cervical triangle. The supraclavicular nerves (medial, intermediate, and lateral), descend to supply the skin overlying the lower half of the posterior cervical triangle, upper chest, and lower third of the anterior cervical triangle. From a clinical standpoint, the main sensory nerve at risk is the great auricular nerve (Figure 5-12) as it ascends over the sternocleidomastoid muscle. Damage to this nerve can result in numbness of the ear, which can be a significant problem for the patient. Identification of the nerve at the time of surgery may be indicated to offer avoidance protection during surgery.

SUMMARY

The head and neck area contains many important anatomic structures that assist in the function of, as well as provide the foundation for, each individual's normal appearance. Proper attention to inoperative technique and details and awareness of the normal and critical anatomic structures allows the dermatologic surgeon to provide the best care to the patient. Cutaneous malignancies may require violation of certain anatomic structures with a resultant residual defect. Preoperative anatomic knowledge and planning will help the dermatologic surgeon achieve the best result and provide appropriate preoperative patient education.

BIBLIOGRAPHY

1. Breisch EA, Greenway HT. *Cutaneous Surgical Anatomy of the Head and Neck* (Grekin, RC, ed). New York, NY: Churchill Livingstone; 1992.
2. Hollinshead, WH. *Anatomy for Surgeons. Vol. I. The Head and Neck,* ed 2. New York, NY: Harper and Row; 1969.
3. *Gray's Anatomy*, British 36th ed. Williams PL, Warwick R, eds. Philadelphia, PA: WB Saunders; 1980.

6

LOCAL ANESTHETICS FOR DERMATOLOGIC SURGERY

David E. Kent, MD

Local anesthetic agents are arguably the most important and frequently used drugs in dermatologic surgery. Proper selection and administration of local anesthetics can relieve pain and anxiety in surgical procedures ranging from skin biopsy and excisions to hair transplantation and liposuction. The purpose of this chapter is to provide the practitioner with a data base on local anesthetics in regard to mechanism of action, basic pharmacology, toxicities, dosage, injection technique, selected peripheral nerve blocks, vasoconstrictor use, bicarbonate buffering, and topical anesthetics. In addition, iontophoresis of local anesthetics, tumescent anesthesia, and EMLA cream (a new topical cream) will be discussed.

Historically, leaves of the coca plant *Erythroxylon coca* were chewed by South American Indian cultures. In 1860, Albert Neimann isolated cocaine. Cocaine's clinical[1,2] application for ophthalmologic procedures such as corneal anesthesia was observed in 1860 by Koller[1,2]. A less toxic compound procaine (an ester derivative of para-aminobenzoic acid [PABA]) was synthesized in 1905. After the amide derivative lidocaine was discovered by Lofgren in 1943, newer amide compounds (mepivacaine, bupivacaine, prilocaine, etidocaine) have been synthesized that offer the physician more potent agents with longer durations of action. Lidocaine, along with these other amide agents, is now the most commonly used local anesthetic.

MECHANISM OF ACTION

To understand how local anesthetics block nerve impulse transmission, a brief review of neuroanatomy and impulse transmission may be helpful. Nerve impulse transmission occurs along a nerve axon.[4,5,6,7] The key structure responsible for this conduction is the cell membrane that surrounds the axon. This membrane is rich in phospholipids and is intercalated with protein complexes. Schwann cells surround peripheral nerves and produce a myelin sheath that insulates the nerve fiber. This myelin sheath is not continuous; rather, there are regularly spaced gaps. These gaps are called Nodes of Ranvier. It is at these gaps or interspaces that the nerve membrane is exposed to its surrounding tissue fluid medium. Through this medium a local anesthetic must diffuse to reach the lipid-rich membrane around the nerve axon. The distance between the Nodes of Ranvier (internodal distance) is directly proportional to axon thickness. The thicker (larger) the axon is, the greater the distance between the nodes. Thus, with smaller nerve axon fibers the distance between nodes is shorter. The narrowest nerve fibers are referred to as delta fibers and are responsible for temperature and pain sensation. These smaller sensory fibers have a higher conduction velocity and are anesthetized before larger nerve fibers that are responsible for motor function. These narrow pain and temperature fibers present proportionally less of a barrier for local anesthetic to diffuse through.

Transmembrane ion channels for both sodium (Na+) and potassium (K+) are located at these nodes of Ranvier. Electrical impulse phenomenon in nerves is based on differential resting concentrations of these ions. When a nerve is at rest there exists a high extracellular sodium and a low intracellular sodium concentration; just the opposite holds true for potassium ions. The cell membrane around the nerve is responsible for maintaining these gradients. Once a nerve is stimulated, the permeability of the membrane to sodium increases by opening sodium channels or "gates." Thus, the resting membrane potential (normally -60 to -90 millivolts) at rest starts to depolarize toward the firing threshold of approximately -50 millivolts. Once the firing threshold is reached, sodium channel permeability blows open, resulting in transmission of a nerve impulse.

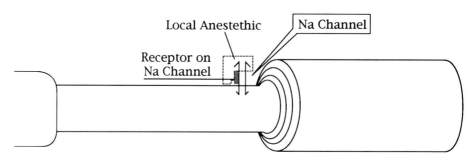

Figure 6.1. Nerve axon surrounded by myelin sheath. Local anesthetic binding to receptor on sodium (Na+) gate blocks Na+ gate, preventing intracellular Na+ movement.

Local anesthetic agents stop nerve impulses by binding to a specific receptor on the axon membrane. This receptor is located at or near the opening of the sodium channel (Figure 6-1). Anesthetic compounds interfere with sodium intracellular movement. Thus, by decreasing the cellular permeability to sodium the action potential is never generated, because the firing threshold is never reached. Another proposed mechanism of action is that local anesthetic agents, being lipid soluble, are absorbed by the lipid-rich membrane, resulting in swelling or expansion of the membrane and corresponding narrowing of the sodium channel (Figure 6-1).

STRUCTURE ACTIVITY RELATIONSHIP

Local anesthetic structure directly influences its activity in regard to potency and duration of action. Local anesthetics have a basic chemical structure: an aromatic portion is connected by either an ester or an amide linkage (the intermediate chain) to the N-terminal amino group.

Aromatic Structure   **Amino Group**

$$COOCH_2 \quad (Ester) \qquad -N \begin{cases} R_1 \\ R_2 \end{cases}$$

$$NHCO \quad (Amide) \qquad -N \begin{cases} R_1 \\ R_2 \end{cases}$$

The aromatic portion is lipophilic and is responsible for its solubility with lipid-rich membranes. Lipid solubility is the single most important determinant of anesthetic potency. Increasing the lipid solubility of a local anesthetic results in increasing local anesthetic potency by allowing the agent to penetrate the membrane more freely. The duration of action of local anesthetic agents is directly related to the degree of protein binding to the interrelated protein complexes. Increasing the size of the intermediate chain increases protein binding to the membrane, thus prolonging duration of action.

CLASSIFICATION

Local anesthetics are classified by their type of linkage to the intermediate group: ester and amide linkages.[5,6,7] Ester compounds are metabolized in the plasma by the enzyme pseudocholinesterase and are excreted in the urine. Cocaine, benzocaine, procaine, tetracaine, and chloroprocaine are examples of ester-linked local anesthetics. Cocaine is a highly effective topical anesthetic with strong vasoconstrictive properties that is frequently used in nasal surgery. Installation into nasal packing via a stock 4% solution is standard. Unfortunately, cocaine has high addictive potential.

Tetracaine is structurally more lipophilic than procaine and more highly protein bound. Thus it is 16 times as potent and has four times the duration of action. It is used for spinal anesthesia as well as for topical anesthesia on mucosal surface membranes.

One of the principal metabolites of the ester group anesthetic is para-aminobenzoic acid (PABA), a known allergen. Consequently, there is documented Type-I allergic reaction potential with ester-type local anesthetics.

Amide local anesthetic agents are metabolized by liver microsomal enzymes and are excreted by the kidney. Lidocaine is the most commonly used local anesthetic. It is available as injectable solution and is active topically on mucous membranes.

Bupivacaine is highly lipid soluble and more strongly protein bound than lidocaine. Both bupivacaine and mepivacaine are more potent and longer-acting than lidocaine. Bupivacaine is four times more potent than lidocaine and has two to three times the duration of action. Etidocaine and prilocaine are two other available amide-linked local anesthetics.

Table 6-1 lists local anesthetic agents, chemical configuration, duration of action, and metabolism site.

TOXIC EFFECTS

Systemic toxic effects of local anesthetics are due primarily to excessive dosage or inadvertent intravascular injection of drug.[8] More than 95% of adverse toxic reactions to local anesthetics are due to excessive dosage. True allergic reactions to local anesthetics are due almost exclusively to ester-linked agents in patients with potential sensitivity to para-aminobenzoic acid. Rare reactions to amide anesthetics have been reported;[9] however, some reported reactions are thought to be related to sulfite preservatives.[10] Systemically, local anesthetics exert an unwanted, exaggerated response that is a pharmacologic characteristic of the drug and not a cytotoxic effect.[8]

Nerve and cardiac muscles have membranes that are susceptible to the pharmacological effects of local anesthetics.[9] The central nervous system is first affected, followed by cardiac conduction tissue and myocardial muscle cells. In the central nervous system (CNS) the balance between inhibitory and facilitory neurons normally exists in the cerebral cortex. When excessive amounts of local anesthetic are given this balance is disrupted, causing initial selective blockade of the inhibitor cortical synapses. This results in uninhibited facilitory neuron activity with excitation of the CNS, manifested by muscular twitching, diplopia, excitement, generalized numbness, dizziness, disorientation, and finally seizure activity. As toxic levels increase, the facilitory neurons are inactivated, resulting in CNS depression and loss of consciousness.[9,11,12,13] At no time does a local anesthetic act as a cortical stimulant; the entire process is one of suppression of electrophysiologic activity.

Regarding the cardiovascular system, local anesthetic dosage at nontoxic levels results in little or no alteration of electrical activity of the heart. As levels approach toxicity, vasodilation occurs and is followed by decreased myocardial contractility. This results in reduced cardiac output, hypotension, and at highly toxic levels, altered cardiac conduction, A-V dissociation, and cardiac arrest.

True allergic reactions to local anesthetics probably make up no more than 1% of all adverse local anesthetic reactions.[15] Glinert and Zachary have provided a discussion of local anesthetic allergy.[16] True allergic reactions are IgE-mediated reactions and are characterized by urticaria, angioedema, bronchospasm, vascular collapse, or shock. Close to 40 cases of presumed IgE-mediated reactions to local anesthetics have been

Table 6.1. Local Anesthetic Agents

Agent Proprietary Name (Trade Name)	Chemical Configuration Aromatic Lipophilic / Intermediate Chain / Amine Hydrophilic	Duration of Action with Epinephrine (in minutes)	Minutes without Epinephrine	Site of Metabolism
(A) Amides				
Lidocaine (Xylocaine)	NHCOCH₂—N(C₂H₅)(C₂H₅), CH₃	60–350	30–100	Liver
Bupivacaine (Marcaine Sensorcaine)	NHCO—(piperidine C₄H₉), CH₃	250–400	120–200	Liver
Mepivacaine (Carbocaine)	NHCO—(piperidine CH₃), CH₃	60–350	30–100	Liver
Etidocaine (Duranest)	NHCOCH—N(C₂H₅)(C₃H₇), CH₃, C₂H₅	240–360	200	Liver
(B) Esters				
Procaine (Novocaine)	H₂N—COOCH₂CH₂—N(C₂H₅)(C₂H₅)	30–90	30	Plasma
Tetracaine	H₉C₄—N(H)—COOCH₂CH₂—N(CH₃)(CH₃)	30	120–240	Plasma
Chloroprocaine (Nesacaine)	H₂N—COOHCH₂—N(C₂H₅)(C₂H₅)	——	30–60	Plasma

reported.[16,17] Over 30% of these were due to lidocaine or other amide-type anesthetic agents.[16]

Preservatives are present in each multidose vial of local anesthetic.[18,19] Parabens and its methyl and propyl derivatives are the most common. Structurally, parabens, which have antibacterial properties, may cross-react immunologically with PABA metabolites of ester-type local anesthetics. Parabens have been judged to be the cause of a small percentage of some patients presumed "caine sensitive."

Paraben-free local anesthetic solutions are commercially available as single-use glass vials. They are intended for one-time use only; any unused solution should be immediately discarded.

A diagnosis of true allergic reactivity is made difficult because of vague or equivocal historical data. To date, there is no specific immunologic test to detect such potential allergic reactions. Review of the literature dealing with local anesthetic skin testing in incremental challenge suggests the following:[15,16,17]

1. Skin testing with local anesthetics may correlate with a history of adverse reaction but may produce systemic adverse reactions, especially with undiluted drugs.
2. Although false-positive skin tests have been reported, most skin-tested patients who subsequently tolerate a local anesthetic have a negative skin test to that drug.
3. False-negative skin tests have not been clearly documented.
4. Incremental challenge beginning with dilute local anesthetics is a safe and effective means of identifying a drug that patients with a history of prior adverse reactions can tolerate.
5. Preservatives in local anesthetics may account for some but not the majority of adverse reactions to local anesthetics. Various protocols for local anesthetic skin testing and incremental challenges have been proposed and are readily used. Any incremental challenge of local anesthetics to patients who are "caine sensitive" should be done so by physicians experienced with allergy testing.

Treatment of toxic levels of local anesthetic is symptomatic, with appropriate airway management, medications, and support personnel. An effective rehearsed emergency plan known to all office personnel is a must for every practitioner and should not be left to chance. Remember, nothing given from a syringe can reverse the respiratory or cardiac arrest induced by an overwhelming dose of local anesthetic.[8]

Systemic toxicity of amide anesthetics has been reported in patients with advanced liver disease.[20] Additional caution should be used when considering larger volumes of amide anesthetics in patients with reduced liver function.

Practical alternatives to local anesthetics exist that allow the dermatologic surgeon to obtain adequate anesthesia when true allergy to local anesthetics is suspected. Injectable physiologic saline may be used to raise a wheal adequate for punch or shave biopsies. Benadryl in a dilution of 10 mg per mL may be used for biopsy or small, simple excisional procedures. If a practitioner suspects true allergy to local anesthetics, then general anesthetics may be considered.

Patients may experience psychogenic reactions based on anxiety and fear of needles and potential pain. Some may even experience true panic attacks. Injection may precipitate vasovagal episodes. Preoperative evaluation by the practitioner may identify patients who will exhibit this behavior. Sometimes direct questions regarding past history of fainting or medication review for antipsychotics will provide a clue. Management of these problems includes Trendelenburg's positioning, supplemental oxygen, maintaining an airway, vital sign monitoring, and, if indicated, epinephrine or noxious stimuli (eg, ammonia inhalants).

DOSAGE

The appropriate dose of local anesthetic agents is dependent on patient size and anesthetic solution concentration. To review, a 1% lidocaine solution contains 10 mg per mL of lidocaine. For adults the maximum recommended dose of lidocaine with epinephrine is 7 mg/kg (eg, for a 70-kg adult 50 cc of a 1% solution or 25 cc of a 2% solution).[21] The maximum dose of lidocaine plain is 4.5 mg/kg (eg, for a 70-kg adult approximately 30 cc of a 1% solution or 15 cc of a 2% solution). For children, the maximum dose is lower, generally one half to one third the adult dose.

When larger volumes of anesthetic are required, a stock solution of 0.5% lidocaine is useful. The maximum recommended single dose of marcaine is up to 225 mg with epinephrine and 175 mg without epinephrine.[22] Marcaine is not recommended for children younger than 12 years of age. The recommended single adult dose of carbocaine for healthy, normal-sized individuals should not exceed 400 mg.[23] This data and that for other anesthetic agents are found in the package insert of each vial. It is advisable for the physician to review this information before initial use. Compounding of local anesthetics (ie, combining marcaine with lidocaine) is a safe technique that permits takes advantage of the best features of each agent (Figure 6-2).[24]

Mixing xylocaine with marcaine provides local anesthesia of rapid onset and long duration. Also, the xylocaine anesthetic effects fall off more abruptly; marcaine seems to wear off more gradually, allowing the patient to adjust better to the return of normal sensation.

VASOCONSTRICTORS

Vasoconstrictors are added to commercially available local anesthetic solutions to produce several desirable effects: (1) constriction of blood vessels in the area of injection reduces rate of absorption of local anesthetic, thus prolonging duration of action; (2) prolonged duration of action reduces the volume of anesthetic solution required; (3) reduced blood loss. Epinephrine is the primary vasoconstrictor in use today. Stock concentrations of epinephrine in commercially available local anesthetics are 1:100,100 and 1:200,000. A solution with 1:100,000 epinephrine has 0.01 mg/mL, and a 1:200,000 solution contains 0.005 mg per mL epinephrine. The recommended maximum dose of epinephrine for 1:100,000 solution (0.01 mg/kg) is 0.20 mg or 20 mL; for a 1:200,000 solution (0.005 mg/kg) it is 0.20 mg or 40 ml.[25]

While commercially available stock concentrations of epinephrine are as mentioned above, one may dilute the concentration of epinephrine to a lower concentration such as 1:400,000 or 1:600,000 and still achieve the desired effects of vasoconstriction.

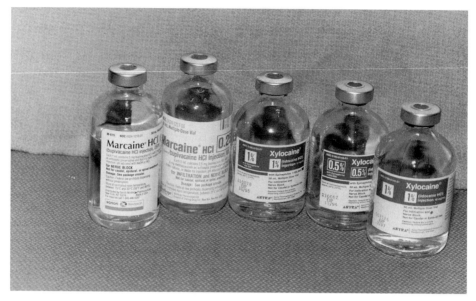

Figure 6.2.   Multidose vials of marcaine 0.5% plain, 0.25% plain, 1% xylocaine with epinephrine, 0.5% xylocaine with epinephrine, 1% xylocaine plain.

For example, to make a solution of 0.5% xylocaine solution with epinephrine concentration of 1:600,000, mix 1 cc of 0.5% xylocaine with epinephrine 1:200,000 (standard stock solution) with 3 cc of 0.5% xylocaine plain. One must allow adequate time for this vasoconstrictive effect to occur. Lidocaine with epinephrine has a pH between 3.3 and 5.5; lidocaine plain (no epinephrine added) is more physiologic, in the range of 5 to 7. Commercially prepared solutions with epinephrine contain preservatives including sodium metabisulfite. Theoretically, sensitivity to bisulfites could manifest itself as an allergic-type reaction.[19]

Neo-cobefrin (levonordefrin) is a vasoconstrictor that is added to commercially available dental carpules of mepivacaine or bupivacaine.[25] Levonordefrin is less potent than epinephrine but has all the same actions. At equally potent doses, Neo-cobefrin stimulates the heart to a greater degree than does epinephrine; thus it has a lower therapeutic index and is not superior to epinephrine.

Epinephrine should be used with extreme caution in patients who are in high-risk groups. These include patients with severe ischemic heart disease, unstable hypertension, peripheral vascular disease, and diabetes. Overdosage or inadvertent intravascular injection of epinephrine containing anesthetics can result in excessively high blood pressure, tachyacardia, and palpitations. As a general rule, local anesthetics containing epinephrine should not be used in digits or in locations with compromised blood flow. This should reduce the risk of ischemic tissue injury.

Various drug-epinephrine–containing solution interactions are possible. Tricyclic antidepressants may potentiate the presser effect of vasoconstrictors.

A potentially life-threatening interaction between the nonselective β-blocker propranolol (inderal) and epinephrine has been reported.[26]

The reported interaction is characterized by a marked hypertensive episode followed quickly by a reflex bradycardia. The six antidotally reported cases share the following similarities: all patients took propranolol (dose 10 to 40 mg/po/bid) and had lidocaine with epinephrine (1:100,000 to 1:200,000) injected in the periorbital region. Further understanding of these antidotal reports awaits controlled clinical evaluation. When performing periorbital surgery on patients taking inderal I suggest using smaller volumes (1 to 3 cc) injected more slowly, instead of rapid infiltration of larger volumes. Also, asking patients if they have ever experienced problems with local anesthetic use may be helpful.

BICARBONATE BUFFERING

In 1987, reports documented the practice of adding exogenous sodium bicarbonate to lidocaine to make local anesthetic injection less painful.[27,28,29] Combining 1 cc of 8.4% sodium bicarbonate to 10 cc of lidocaine with epinephrine raises the pH toward physiologic pH and may actually reduce the sting of injection.

If larger volumes are required, a 1% lidocaine with epinephrine and 80 mEq/L sodium bicarbonate solution can be prepared by adding 5.0 mL of 7.5% sodium bicarbonate solution (Lyphomed or American Regent Labs) or 4.5 mL of 8.4% solution and adding this to a 50-mL multidose vial of 1% solution.[30] Because of potential attenuation of the epinephrine effect, the buffered anesthetic solution should be discarded within one week of preparation.[31]

TECHNIQUE

Once the appropriate local anesthetic has been selected, it is ready to be administered. Smaller-gauge needles (27–30 gauge) that are 1/2 inch to 1 1/2 inches in length combined with disposable syringes (3 to 12 cc) are routinely used. Some physicians use dental syringes with disposable cartridges of lidocaine 2% with epinephrine, or carbocaine or marcaine. While the advantages of quick assembly and utilization are evident, one cannot easily aspirate through the syringes adequately to test for intravascular injection (Figure 6-3).

In general, gently angulated needle placement and a slow delivery of anesthetic solution, with the skin stretched taut, causes less pain than does a tangential needle jab with rapid infiltration. Rapid infiltration of local anesthetic produces tissue distention and significant discomfort. On the central part of the face, entering the skin via a follicular orifice may produce less pain.

After initially placing a few drops of local anesthetic intradermally, a 2- to 10-second pause will allow this area to become anesthetized adequately. More anesthetic may then be injected to raise a small intradermal wheal with reduced pain. As the wheal expands, the needle may be removed and reinserted through the already anesthetized tissue and advanced while the anesthetic is slowly infiltrated. This minimizes the number of uncomfortable needle sticks experienced by the patient. Aspiration while advancing the needle (backward pull of the syringe plunger during needle advancement), especially in highly vascularized areas, greatly reduces the chance of an intravascular injection.

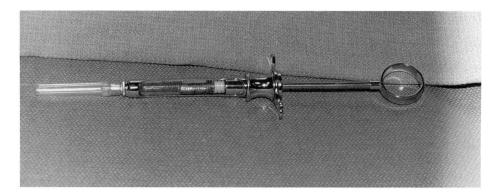

Figure 6.3. Dental syringe, carpule with 2% xylocaine with epinephrine 1:100000, 30-gauge one-inch dental needle.

Gentle rubbing and massage of the area that has been anesthetized will speed the diffusion of the local anesthetic into the intended tissues.

Local anesthetic agents may be used for direct infiltration of the planned surgical area or by nerve block. For planned excisional surgery, use of a sterile gentian violet marking pen to draw the planned excision on the skin surface provides a good outline for placement of local anesthetic. After first placing a wheal of anesthetic, the needle is advanced to the mid or deeper portion of the reticular dermis. Needle placement should be at the deeper portion of the reticular dermis. Injecting directly through a malignant lesion may potentially transfer malignant cells, so this practice should be avoided. Although unlikely, transfer of malignant cells by "spearing" small pieces with a needle theoretically could occur. This would seem more likely if larger-caliber needles were used (eg, 25 gauge instead of 30 gauge).

Important points to remember before beginning any dermatologic surgical procedure include (1) paying attention to the patient's physical comfort and checking whether he or she has utilized the restroom before the procedure; (2) when working on the face, protecting the patient's eyes from bright surgical lights when possible; (3) informing the patient of what you are planning to do and when to anticipate any discomfort; (4) informing the patient that the anesthetic will eliminate his or her pain but not sensations of pulling or pressure, and that these sensations are generally well tolerated. These simple steps tend to reduce the patient's fears and anxieties and make the patient feel safe and relaxed. A calm, relaxed patient bleeds less, requires less local anesthetic, and is more cooperative.

NERVE BLOCK OF THE HEAD AND NECK

Nerve Supply to the Head and Neck

An understanding of the sensory supply to the head and neck is mandatory when performing nerve block anesthesia. The principal sensory supply of the face is via the sensory fibers of the trigeminal nerve. The intracranial and extracranial course of the trigeminal nerve are well documented[32,33,34] (see Chapter 5 Figs. 5-1a and 5-1b).

The ophthalmic division has five branches: supraorbital, supratrochlear, infratrochlear, external nasal, and lacrimal nerves. The supraorbital nerve exists through the supraorbital notch, a readily palpable, bony landmark along the supraorbital ridge. It is located at the midpupillarly position approximately 2.5 cm lateral of midline. A vertically constructed plumb line connects this nerve with the exit points of the infraorbital nerve via the infraorbital foramen, and the mental nerve via the mental foramen. The supratrochlear, infratrochlear, and lacrimal branches do not have any bony landmarks (Figure 6-4). The supratrochlear nerve exits with the same named vessels at the upper medial angle of the orbit under the frontalis and orbicularis oculi muscles and supplies the skin in the region of the glabella. The infratrochlear nerve appears just above the medial angle of the eye and supplies the skin of the upper eyelid and upper portion of the nasal root. The external nasal nerve exits at the junction of the nasal bone and the upper lateral nasal cartilages to supply innervation to the nasal tip. The lacrimal branch innervates the skin on the lateral portion of the upper eyelid.

The maxillary division of the trigeminal nerve is composed of the infraorbital, zygomaticofacial, and zygomaticotemporal branches. The infraorbital nerve exits from the infraorbital foramen, a bony landmark approximately 1 cm inferior to the bony orbital rim and supplies the upper lip, wing of the nose, upper part of the cheek, and

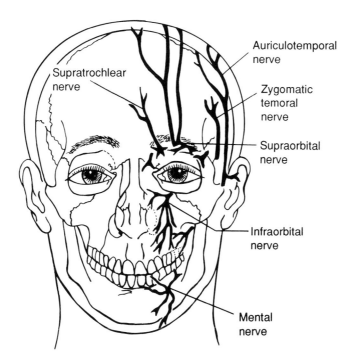

Figure 6.4. Sensory nerve supply to the face. Note a verticle plumb line connects the supraorbital, intraorbital, and mental foramen. The supraorbital foramen is located 2.5 cm away from midline. Ideally, the sequence of a supraorbital nerve block may run from the medial aspect of the brow in a lateral direction.

lower eyelid. The zygomaticofacial nerve supplies the skin over the zygomatic arch. The zygomaticotemporal nerve supplies a small area in the anterior temporal region.

The cutaneous branches of the mandibular nerve are the auriculotemporal, the buccal, and the mental nerves. The auriculotemporal nerve is located just anterior to the tragus and turns upward in close relation to the superficial temporal artery to supply the upper portion of the ear and the posterior portion of the temporal region.

The lesser occipital nerve crosses the upper sternocleidomastoid to supply the skin of the lower lateral scalp posterior to the external ear (Figure 6-5).

The great auricular nerve runs anterior superiorly to supply the skin over the mandibular angle and posterior pinna. The transverse cutaneous nerve crosses the sternocleidomastoid transversely at about its midpoint to supply the skin over the anterior triangle of the neck.

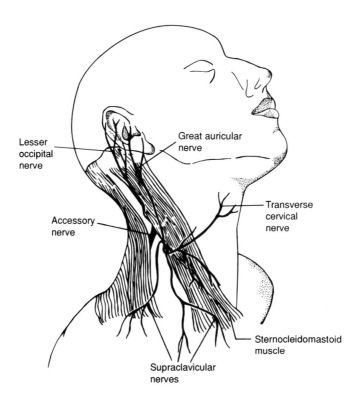

Figure 6.5. Sensory nerve supply to the neck and a portion of the ear. Both the great auricular and lesser occipital nerves are anesthetized as part of a "ring block" anesthesia of the auricle. The lateral neck may be anesthetized via a local block of the transverse cervical, great auricular, and supraclavicular nerves as they exit from the posterior border of the midportion of the sternocleidomastoid muscle dividing the anterior and posterior triangles of the neck. Note the relatively unprotected motor spiral accessory nerve superior to the site for the local neck block.

The buccal nerve emerges from under the anterior border of the masseter and runs downward and forward to supply the skin of the lower part of the cheek. The mental nerve supplies the skin of the chin and lower lip.

The ear receives its sensory innervation by branches of trigeminal, facial, glossopharyngeal, and vagus cranial nerves and the sensory branches of the cervical plexus. The areas of the scalp are supplied by the supraorbital and supratrochlear nerves anteriorly, the zygomaticotemporal, auriculotemporal, and posterior auricular nerves laterally, and the lesser occipital and greater occipital nerves posteriorly. These nerves form a ring about the scalp at about the level of the glabella region.

The neck is superficially divided into anterior and posterior cervical triangles with the sternocleidomastoid muscle being the divider, the mandible and clavicle serving as superior and inferior boundaries. The cutaneous branches of the cervical plexus emerge from the posterior triangle at the posterior border of the sternocleidomastoid and turn anteriorly across the muscle.

Nerve Block Anesthesia

To obtain nerve block anesthesia, the anesthetic must reach the nerve early in its course to the area targeted. The nerve proper should not be injected, as this may injure the nerve and result in prolonged paresthesias or neuroma formation. Instead, one should "bathe" the nerve proper with anesthetic. If doubt exists that the needle is in a nerve, withdraw the needle several millimeters and inject. Aspiration during needle advancement should prevent inadvertent intravascular injection. Finally, the patient should be told that paresthesias might be experienced during administration of the anesthetic.

Supraorbital Forehead and Frontal Scalp Block; Scalp Block

To obtain sensory block of the forehead, the supraorbital and supratrochlear nerves must be anesthetized. A simple technique is to inject local anesthetic along the superior portion of the eyebrow line. First, raise a small wheal just lateral of midline at the upper edge of the eyebrow. Next, directing the needle laterally in the superficial subcutaneous fat, bathe the supratrochlear, and superorbital nerves in 2 to 3 cc mL of local anesthetic (Figure 6-4). Injecting directly into the supraorbital foramen may injure the nerve and should be avoided. "Massaging" the skin after injection and taping a gauze sponge over the injection site, producing slight pressure, will speed the onset of anesthesia.

After waiting 5 to 10 minutes for the nerve block to take, local reinforcements of anesthetic with epinephrine at the surgery site will aid in hemostasis. The operator must allow adequate time for the local anesthetic to take effect.

The scalp can be completely anesthetized by injecting a ring of anesthesia circumferentially above the level of the glabella. Small scalp lesions may not require field block anesthesia but a simple ring block by merely injecting the proposed area of incision site with local anesthetic. Table 6-2 summarizes various nerve blocks useful for the head and neck. Chapter 5 (page 88) delineates the sensory divisions of the trigeminal nerve as do figs. 5-1a and 5-1b.

Table 6.2. Selected Nerve Blocks of the Head and Neck

Expected Area of Anesthesia	Nerve Block
Scalp (A) Frontal	Supraorbital n.
	Supratrochlear n.
(B) Lateral	Zygometicotemporal n.
	Auriculotemporal n.
	Lesser occipital n.
(C) Posterior	Greater occipital n.
	Lesser occipital n.
Forehead	Supraorbital n.
	Supratrochlear n.
Mid-Cheek, Upper lip	Infraorbital n.
Nasal Sidewall	Infraorbital n.
	Infratrochlear n.
Chin, Lower lip	Mental n.
Lateral Neck	Cutaneous branches of cervical plexus (C2, C3, C4)

Infraorbital Cheek and Lip Block

To obtain sensory block of the middle third of the face including the upper lip, the infraorbital and infratrochlear nerves must be anesthetized. The infraorbital nerve may be blocked by either an extraoral or an intraoral approach. The intraoral approach is less painful. First, a topical anesthetic is placed on the mucous membrane at the gum cheek reflection to reduce initial needle-stick sting. With one finger over the infraorbital foramen (5 mm below the inferior margin of the orbit), elevate the lip with the gloved thumb and second finger. The needle is inserted to a depth of several millimeters, and a few drops of anesthetic are injected. The needle is then directed toward the foramen and the nerve rootlets are bathed with 2 to 3 mL of anesthetic. With the extraoral approach, the needle is inserted through the skin at a point overlying the infraorbital foramen, which is found approximately 2.5 cm below the eyelid margin; a few drops of anesthetic are placed intradermally to anesthetize the immediate skin area. The needle is carefully advanced deeper toward the foramen, and the nerve rootlets are again "bathed" with a similar volume of anesthetic. The infratrochlear nerve is blocked at its exit point along the lateral nasal root.

Mental Lip and Chin Block

To obtain sensory block of the chin and lower lip, anesthetize the mental nerve. Again, both the extraoral and intraoral approaches are available, but the intraoral approach produces less pain. The intraoral approach for the mental nerve (located in the height of the body of the mandible between the premolars) is identical to the infraorbital nerve except the lower lip is elevated, exposing the gum cheek reflection, and the same steps are followed.

Great Auricular and Ring Ear Block

The entire ear can be anesthetized by injecting local anesthetic around the auricle and into the conchal bowl to block the greater auricular, lesser occipital, auriculotemporal, and auricular branches of the vagus nerve. Beginning inferiorly to the lobule and directing the injection posteriorly and superiorly toward the mastoid and moving superiorly, anesthetize the posterior ear. Doing the similar technique along the preauricular areas will "ring" the ear successfully.

Neck Block

The cutaneous branches of the cervical plexus (the transverse cervicle, supraclavicular, and great auricular nerves) emerge from the posterior border in the midportion of the sternocleidomastoid muscle to provide sensory innervation to the lateral neck. Superior to this the lesser occipital nerve exits, providing sensory innervation more superiorly, including a portion of the ear. A local block via infiltration of the exit point of the cutaneous branches of this cervical plexus will provide local anesthesia of the lateral neck (Figure 6-5). Note the position of the spinal accessory nerve, which provides innervation for motor elevation of the trapezius muscle. Aspiration is critical when anesthetizing the skin and soft tissues of the neck. Large vessels may act as inadvertent targets, especially in elderly patients.

Nasal Block

Anesthesia of the external nose requires a combination of nerve blocks and local field block infiltration. The infraorbital nerves are blocked bilaterally as described and the infratrochlear nerves are blocked at the lateral nasal root area. The external nasal nerve supplying the nasal tip is blocked where it exits at the junction of the upper lateral nasal cartilages and the distal nasal base.

The base of the columella is supplied by the anterior spinous nerve and may be anesthetized directly through the skin or via an intraoral approach.

Digital Block for Finger or Toe

Digital block of the finger or toe provides local anesthesia of the digit and the distal nail area. Plain 1% lidocaine is used at the base of the digit to anesthetize the lateral digital nerves. While 2% lidocaine plain can also be used, it may have less of a duration of action, as it causes more vasodilation. In any case, large volumes of local anesthesia should be avoided so as not to impede venous return. With a 30-gauge, one-inch needle, a small amount of 1% lidocaine plain is injected at the base of the digit laterally to block the inferior and superior digital nerves. This process is repeated on the opposite lateral side, again superficial to the periosteum at the base of the digit. Full bilateral blockade is required to provide complete digital anesthesia.

TOPICAL ANESTHETICS

Topical anesthetic agents for intact glabrous skin may reduce the discomfort from needle sticks. Simple agents that may be of benefit include ice cubes and cryoanesthetics such as ethyl chloride and the Freon-containing refrigerant sprays: Frigederm, Fluorethyl, and others. Should these cold refrigerant spray products be used, the areas not treated must be protected; short spray times are preferred to reduce the likelihood of cryoinjury to the soft tissues. Surface-active topical anesthetics are very effective on mucosal surfaces. They should not be injected or applied in large volumes owing to rapid absorption. Other topical local anesthetic agents include a variety of products of the previously mentioned local anesthetic agents. These agents may be employed as ointments, jellies, and spray products.

For example, lidocaine is available for topical uses as a 2% viscous jelly, a 2.5% to 5% ointment, and a 4% topical solution. Benzocaine 20% (Hurricane) can also be used, topically or in a topical aerosol spray, on mucosal surfaces as a topical anesthetic. In our practice the use of Hurricane or lidocaine intraorally on the mucosa before the intraoral approach for an infraorbital or mental nerve block allows elimination of the pain from the initial needle contact with the mucosa, thus easing the patient's anxiety.

EMLA cream is a new topical anesthetic intended for use on intact glaberous skin.[38] It is a eutectic mixture of lidocaine 2.5% and prilocaine 2.5%. These two anesthetics, when mixed with the appropriate compounding oils and water emulsion, penetrate observably through cornified skin. Studies document reduced painful stimulus from needle pinprick when EMLA cream is applied 90–120 minutes under occlusion before painful stimulus.

Applications for use of EMLA cream include superficial surgery, split-thickness skin graft harvesting, venapuncture, laser surgery, and debridement of superficial wounds.[40,41,42,43] EMLA cream must be applied to the skin in a thick layer, occluded, and left in place for 90–120 minutes to work. It is especially helpful for curetting off molluscum in children. It also may be useful topically before needle infiltration with a local anesthetic.

The use of topical ocular anesthetics makes many procedures in ophthalmologic and dermatologic surgery possible. Commonly used topical ocular anesthetics include tetracaine (pontocaine) and proparacaine (opthaine). Absorption across these mucosal surfaces is very rapid.[35] For example, within 30 minutes after ocular installation of radioactive corticosteroid, only 1.6% of that radioactive steroid remains in the eye area, the rest having crossed the conjunctiva and become distributed throughout the body.[36] For example, 100 mg of tetracaine (only 5 mL of a 2% solution) is a potential lethal dose. The rate of absorption across mucous membranes is not generally appreciated, but is actually 5–10 times greater than the rate of absorption from an equal volume of fluid injected subcutaneously or intramuscularly.[37] Increasing the concentration of topical anesthetics beyond the commonly used concentration (.05% proparacaine, .5% tetracaine) does not enhance onset or duration of anesthesia, instead resulting mainly in increased systemic toxicity. Effective corneal and conjunctival anesthesia may be achieved within 1 to 2 minutes after 2 to 3 drops topically of proparacaine or tetracaine and lasts for 10 to 15 minutes. Installation may be repeated as necessary to prolong anesthesia. An initial burning sensation (worse with tetracaine) may be followed by a peculiar numb sensation that causes some patients to rub their eyes in annoyance. The patient should therefore be cautioned.

Allergy to topical anesthetics is not common but can be severe. Tetracaine allergy may cause swollen, irritated, reddened, itching eyelids that persist for days after initial evaluation. Proparacaine allergy presents itself differently. Within 10 minutes after installation epithelial stippling and slight corneal edema appear, which may result in sufficient blurring of vision to make walking difficult. The conjunctiva becomes puffy and reddened but the lids are not swollen as in typical allergy. Pain and tearing may persist for hours.

Iontophoresis is the process of active transport of charged ions across a membrane by means of an electric current.[44] Local anesthetic solutions containing 4% lidocaine have been administered effectively by iontophoresis. Iontophoresis of local anesthetic is especially helpful for the sole of the foot or before nerve blocks in apprehensive patients.

TUMESCENT ANESTHESIA

Tumescent anesthesia is a technique using large volumes of very dilute lidocaine with epinephrine and is most frequently applied in liposuction[45,46]. This technique has revolutionized liposuction, allowing the procedure to be better performed with fewer risks. Broader roles for dilute solutions of lidocaine and epinephrine in areas such as hair transplantation and scalp reduction (ie, 50 to 100 mL), dermabrasion, and other cutaneous surgical procedures are now being explored and evaluated[47].

SUMMARY

Local anesthetics are an integral part of dermatologic surgery. Correct selection, dosage, and use will "set the stage" for uneventful surgical procedures. Pain during or after surgery is a fear all patients have. Establishing good communication between patient and physician before surgery, combined with proper local anesthetic use, will relieve pain and anxiety for all involved.

REFERENCES

1. McAuley JE. The early development of local anesthesia. *Br Dent J.* 121:139–141, 1966.
2. Fink BR. Leaves and needles: The introduction of surgical local anesthesia. *Anesthesiology.* 63:77–83, 1985.
3. Wildsmith JA, Strichartz ER. Local anesthetic drugs: An historical perspective. *Br J Anesthesiol.* 56:937–939, 1984.
4. Covino BG. Local anesthesia. *N Eng J Med.* 286:975–983, 1972.
5. Truant AP, Takman B. Differential physio-chemical and neuropharmacologic properties of local anesthetic agents. *Anesthesiology.* 38:478–484, 1969.
6. Covino BG. New developments in the field of local anesthetics and the scientific basis for their clinical use. *Acta Anesthesiol Scand.* 26:242–249, 1982.
7. Reynolds F. The pharmacology of local anesthetic drugs. In: Churchill Davidson HC, ed. *A Practice of Anesthesia.* Chicago, IL: Yearbook Medical Publishers; 830–855, 1984.
8. Adrian J. Naraghim: Local anesthetics: Who should give them? *South Med J.* 78:1219–1223, 1985.
9. Adrian J. Local anesthetic toxicity. *Anesthesiol Rev.* 10:11–15, 1983.
10. Glinert RJ, Zachary CB. Local anesthetic allergy—its recognition and avoidance. *J Dermatol Surg Oncol.* 17:491–496, 1991.
11. Wagmen IH, Dejong RH, Prince OQ. Effects of lidocaine on the central nervous system. *Anesthesiology.* 28:155–172, 1967.

12. Tanaka K, Yamajak M. Blocking of cortical inhibitory synapses by intravenous lidocaine. *Nature*. 209:207–208, 1966.

13. Dejong RH, Robies R, Crobin RW. Central actions of lidocaine-synaptic transmission. *Anesthesiology*. 30:19–20, 1969.

14. Bigger JT, Jr, Matel WJ. Effect of lidocaine in the electrophysiological properties of ventricular muscle and Purkinje fibers. *J Clin Invest*. 49:63–77, 1970.

15. Giovannitti JA, Bennett CR. Assessment of allergy to local anesthetics. *JAMA*. 98:701–706, 1979.

16. Schatz M. Skin testing and incremental challenge in the evaluation of adverse reactions. *J Allergy Clin Immunol*. 74:600–616, 1984.

17. Kennedy KS, Cave RH. Anaphylactic reaction to lidocaine. *Arch Otolaryngol Head Neck Surg*. 112:671–673, 1986.

18. Luebke NH, Walker JA. Discussion of sensitivity to preservatives in anesthetics. *J Am Dent Assoc*. 97:656–657, 1978.

19. Schwartz HJ, Sherth T. Bisulfite sensitivity manifesting as allergy to local dental anesthesia. *J Allergy Clin Immunol*. 75:525–527, 1985.

20. Selden R, Sasahara A. Central nervous system toxicity induced by lidocaine: Report of a case in a patient with liver disease. *JAMA*. 202:908–909, 1967.

21. Package insert. Xylocaine. Astra Pharmaceuticals. Westborough, MA, 1992.

22. Package insert. Marcaine. Winthrop Pharmaceuticals, New York, NY, 1993.

23. Package insert. Carbocaine. Winthrop Pharmaceuticals, New York, NY, 1988.

24. Moore DC. Does compounding of local anesthetic agents increase their toxicity in humans? *Anest Analg*. 51:579–585, 1972.

25. New York Heart Association. Report of the special committee of the New York Heart Association, Inc, on the use of epinephrine in connection with procaine in dental procedures. *J Am Dent Assoc*. 50:108–113, 1955.

26. Foster CA, Aston SJ. Propranolol-epinephrine interaction: a potential disaster. *Plastic Reconst Surg*. 72:74–78, 1983.

27. Mckay W, Morris RM, Mushlin P. Sodium bicarbonate attenuates pain on skin infiltration with lidocaine, with or without epinephrine. *Anesthesiol Ann*. 66:572–574, 1987.

28. Korbson GA, Hurley DP, Williams GS. Ph adjusted lidocaine does not "sting." *Anesthesiology*. 66:855–856, 1987.

29. Christopher RS, Buchanan RN, Begelia K, Schwartz S. Pain reduction in local anesthetic administration through Ph buffering. *Ann Emerg Med*. 17:117–120, 1988.

30. Stewart JH, Cole GW, Kelin JS. Neutralized lidocaine with epinephrine for local anesthesia—II. *J Dermatol Surg Oncol*. 16:842–845, 1990.

31. Stewart JH, Cole GW, Kelin JA. Neutralized lidocaine for local anesthesia. *J Dermatol Surg Oncol*. 16:1081–1083, 1989.

32. Breisch EA, Greenway HT, Jr. *Cutaneous Surgical Anatomy of the Head and Neck*. New York, NY: Churchill Livingstone; 1992:1–108.

33. Woodburne RT. *Essentials of Human Anatomy*. New York, Oxford University Press Inc; 1968; 197–198, 219–222.

34. Panje WR. Local anesthesia of the face. *J Dermatol Surg Oncol*. 5:312–315, 1979.

35. Adrian J, Campbell D. Fatalities following topical application of local anesthetics to mucous membranes. *JAMA*. 162:1527–1529, 1956.

36. Jones RG, Stiles JF. The penetration of cortisol into normal and pathologic rabbit eyes. *Am J Ophthalmol*. 56:84–88, 1963.

37. Havener W. Ocular therapeutics. In: Peyman GA, Sanders DR, Goldberg ME. *Principles and Practice of Ophthalmology*, 1st ed. Philadelphia, PA: Saunders; 1980:743–744.

38. Lycka BA. EMLA. A new and effective topical anesthetic. *J Dermatol Surg Oncol*. 18:859–862, 1992.

39. Juhlin L, Evers H. EMLA: A new topical anesthetic. In: Callen JP, Dohl MV, Galitz LE, Greenway HT, Jr., Schachner LA, eds. *Advances in Dermatology, Vol. 5.* Chicago, IL: Year Book; 1990:75–91.

40. Der Waard-Van DK, Spek FB, Oranje AO, Lilleborg S, Hop WC, Stolz E. Treatment of molluscum contagiosum using a lidocaine/prilocaine cream (EMLA) for analgesia. *J Am Acad Dermatol.* 23:685–91, 1990.

41. Juhlin L, Evers H, Brobeg F. A lidocaine/prilocaine cream for superficial skin surgery and painful lesions. *Acta Derm Venerol.* 60:544–546, 1980.

42. Halperin DL, Koren G, Attins D, et al. Topical skin anesthesia for venous, subcutaneous drug reservoir and lumbar punctures in children. *Pediatrics.* 84:281–284, 1989.

43. Arendt-Nielsen L, Bjerring P. Laser induced pain for evaluation of local anesthesia: A comparison of topical application (EMLA) and local injection (lidocaine). *Anesthesia.* 67:115–123, 1988.

44. Maloney M, Bezzant JL, Stephen RL, Petelenz TJ. Iontopheretic administration of lidocaine anesthesia in office practice. *J Dermatol Surg Oncol.* 18:937–940, 1992.

45. Klein JA. Anesthesia for liposuction in dermatologic surgery. *J Dermatol Surg Oncol.* 14:1124–1132, 1988.

46. Klein JA. Tumescent technique for regional anesthesia permits lidocaine doses of 35 mg/kg for liposuction. *J Dermatol Surg Oncol.* 16:248–263, 1990.

47. Coleman WP III, Kelin JA. The tumescent anesthetic technique for scalp surgery, dermabrasion, and soft tissue reconstruction. *J Dermatol Surg Oncol.* 18:130–135, 1992.

7

WOUND HEALING AND DRESSINGS

D.J. Papadopoulos, MD

INTRODUCTION

From prehistoric times through antiquity and into the modern era, humans have paid particular attention and devoted much of their time toward the managements of wounds. Prehistoric artifacts, as well as numerous museum pieces, depict scenes of the applications of different dressings on the wounded, predominantly in times of warfare, but also in times of peace. We know that certain societies throughout the ancient world created surgical wounds and subsequently provided care for these wounds in an attempt to rid the afflicted individual of a variety of maladies from mental illness to venous varicosities. Indeed, skulls from ancient pre-Columbian societies show multiple trepanations in different stages of *healing*.[1] During these times, common bleeding was dealt with through the use of masticated herbs and simple, tourniquetlike pressure dressings.

The ancient Egyptians, probably through the immense experience gained as a result of mummification procedures, were using linen strips and adhesive plasters as wound dressings.[2] As the art of healing and medicine progressed, and as physicians were increasingly asked to accompany armies into battle, so did their capacity to provide care for wounds. Achilles, besides being a nearly immortal warrior during the siege of Troy in Greek legend, was also known to provide medical care. On the bowl of Sosias at the Staatliche Museum in Berlin, he is depicted bandaging the wounds of his comrade, Patroclus.[1]

Linen dressings, after thousands of years, eventually gave way to gauze dressings in the late 19th century as popularized by Gamgee.[3] With the advent of synthetic dressings in the middle of this century, and with the explosion of knowledge pertaining to wound healing on a macroscopic as well as microscopic level over the past 20 years, we have now reached an era of being able to modify the events of wound healing, and in the near future we will be in a position to intervene in types of injury previously considered unmanageable. In this chapter, I will attempt to discuss certain fundamental aspects of wound healing and the management of surgically created cutaneous wounds by appropriate dressing techniques.

WOUND HEALING

Traditionally, we have been taught that wound healing proceeds through three classic phases—the inflammatory, reconstructive, and remodeling phases. There are excellent reviews describing in great detail the phases of wound healing.[4,5,6] I will briefly review some of the basic concepts of these three phases.

Inflammatory Phase (First Week after Wounding)

Within seconds after a wound is established, there is an immediate vasoconstriction that lasts approximately 5–10 minutes, followed by subsequent vasodilation. Platelets initially adhere to the cut surfaces of blood vessels and aggregate to form a hemostatic plug. These platelets are also responsible for releasing ADP, vasoactive substances, chemoattractants, growth factors, and proteases that stimulate the alternative complement pathway. These factors, either by themselves or through their role in stimulating other factors, guide the inflammatory phase through the important processes of temporarily coapting the wound edges, cross-linking fibronectin, and laying down a provisional matrix upon which fibroblast and epithelial cells can begin to adhere.

Immediately after wounding, as the clot is being established, polymorphonuclear leukocytes and macrophages are chemoattracted to the wound. Polymorphonuclear leukocytes are the predominant cell type within the first two days after wounding. Their role is mainly one of phagocytosis, and their presence is not absolutely mandatory for wound healing to proceed at a normal rate.[7] The presence and proper function of the macrophage, however, is critical to the normal progression of wound healing.[8] Its functions include killing of bacteria, foreign-body debridement, digestion of devitalized collagen, and influence on fibroblasts and endothelial cells to promote granulation tissue formation. Toward the end of the inflammatory phase (the fifth or sixth day after wounding), there is an influx of lymphocytes, which may, along with macrophages, secrete chemotactic factors that stimulate fibroblast proliferation and collagen deposition.

Reconstructive Phase (Fourth Day to Fourteenth Day)

The onset of this phase overlaps with the inflammatory phase; indeed, all the phases of wound healing should be considered as a continuum. The hallmarks of this phase are granulation-tissue formation and reepithelialization. For granulation to occur, there must initially be an intense proliferation of fibroblasts and capillaries.

These, along with macrophages, become imbedded in fibrin, fibronectin, Types-III and -I collagen, and hyaluronic acid. This mixture of cellular and matrix components represents granulation tissue. The matrix components are in large part produced by fibroblasts.

The second prominent feature of this phase is resurfacing of the wound. This process is known as epithelialization when the resurfacing emanates from the wound edges and adnexal structures from below, or as epidermization when the process involves resurfacing without the reformation of glandular or follicular structures.

The act of resurfacing occurs almost instantly after wounding, and the rate at which it proceeds is in large part controlled by local factors, including the establishment of a provisional matrix, the water content of the wound bed,[9] serum factors such as epibolin, epidermal growth factor (EGF), and platelet-derived growth factor (PDGF), as well as epidermally derived chalone inhibition after wounding. Chalones normally function to inhibit epidermal proliferation and migration. Wounding may inhibit chalone production.

It is important to note that resurfacing ceases after the wound is covered and there is contact of apposing epidermal migratory sheets. This is known as contact inhibition. The new epidermis has few rete ridges and its dermal attachment is weak, resulting in easy blistering and detachment. In addition, especially in full-thickness wounds, melanocyte repopulation and function is incomplete. During the latter part of the reconstructive phase, wound contraction takes on a significant role in determining the final appearance of the healed wound. This phenomenon is in large part caused by myofibroblasts (transformed fibroblasts), which are an integral part of granulation tissue. This cell has contractile and migratory capabilities as a result of possessing actin-like microfilaments in its cytoplasm parallel to its long axis.[10]

During the reconstructive phase, collagen production and remodeling is predominantly controlled by fibroblasts. Initially, Type-III collagen is laid out on a framework of fibronectin,[11] but as the cicatrix matures, Type-I collagen predominates. Likewise, there is a difference in the glycosoaminoglycan milieu of the wound based on time after wounding, with hyaluronic acid the most prominent component in the early stages. Hyaluronic acid, because of its high water content, may facilitate cell migration. As wound coverage is accomplished, chondroitin-4-sulfate, dermatan sulfate, and heparin sulfate predominate, probably as a result of the relative need for more stabilization of cell-fibronectin adherence.[12,13,14,15]

Remodeling Phase (Two Weeks to One Year)

From the onset of matrix formation and the generation of granulation tissue in the previous two phases, there is a constant process of remodeling of the composition and structure of these two components. This remodeling leads to the eventual dissolution of granulation tissue, the elimination of most fibronectin from the matrix, and gradual accumulation of large bundles of Type-I collagen. Despite the replacement of granulation tissue by collagen, wounds gain tensile strength very slowly, and indeed have gained only about 20% of their final strength by the third week. The maximum tensile strength of a scar approaches 70–80% of intact skin.[16]

Wound contraction is also an important component of the remodeling phase. As mentioned before, contraction is mediated largely by the specialized connections of myofibroblasts to the extracellular matrix.[17,18] Decrease in the size of the wound ultimately minimizes the area to be repaired and begins at about seven to eight days after wounding, but does not become clinically apparent until the 14th day. The depth of wounding tends to dictate whether contraction will occur. Specifically, superficial wounds, where the injury has depths into the papillary dermis, contract very little, if at all. It is possible that the presence of reticular dermis may be an important factor in inhibiting contraction; wounds devoid of reticular dermis contract significantly. The critical component, once again, may be the myofibroblast, which is found in the reticular dermis and is probably activated by full-thickness injury.[19]

Vascularization tends to diminish as remodeling progresses. In the very early stages of wound healing, hypoxic conditions that exist in the wound stimulate the production of macrophage-derived angiogenesis factor, which leads to neovascularization.[20,21] As blood flow and tissue oxygenation increase, this angiogenic factor decreases, with resultant decreases in new vessel formation and subsequently reabsorption of existing vessels. Thus clinically, with time, scars tend to be relatively avascular in their appearance.

FACTORS AFFECTING WOUND HEALING

There are many factors that influence either one, two, or all three phases of wound healing. These factors have as a direct consequence a positive or negative impact on the healing wound. For practical purposes I will divide these factors into systemic factors and local factors.

Systemic Factors Affecting Wound Healing

Age

Keratinocytes derived from neonates have much greater in vitro duration of life and proliferative capacity than those derived from adults.[22,23] Studies on animals and humans have shown that aging is accompanied by decreases in the inflammatory and proliferative responses, and by delays in angiogenesis, re-epithelialization, and remodeling.[24] Thus, from a clinical point of view, we must exercise prudence when considering suture placement, type of suture used, time of suture removal, adjunctive antibiotic therapy based on location of the wound, and advice we give our patients as to when they can resume normal physical activity.

Nutrition

Relative protein and carbohydrate deficiency may delay fibroplasia and matrix formation and impair wound remodeling. This may lead to decreased tensile strength. Furthermore, during these deficiency states, cellular and humoral immune responses are impaired, leading to a greatly increased possibility of secondary infection.[25]

Vitamin deficiencies have been associated with delayed wound healing. Vitamin A deficiency leads to decreased rates of epithelialization, decreased collagen synthesis, and increased risk of secondary infection. Vitamin C deficiency, although rare in the United States, could lead to wound dehiscence as a result of the critical role played by this molecule in the hydroxylation of proline and lysine residues during collagen synthesis. Underhydroxylated collagen is unstable and subject to collagenolysis. Vitamin K deficiency results in hematoma formation due to diminished production of essential clotting factors (II, VII, IX, X). This deficiency also results in the production of faulty clots that cannot sustain collagen and matrix support.[25] Zinc deficiency may be associated with a host of abnormalities, including decreased immune response, decreased collagen synthesis, and disruption of remodeling of the wound.[26]

In the absence of a tissue vitamin or trace-element deficiency state, the routine administration of supplemental vitamins does not enhance wound healing significantly. The only exception to this may be the concurrent administration of vitamin A to individuals who have been on long-term corticosteroids and who have experienced poor wound healing in the past.[27]

Oxygenation

Tissue ischemia and subsequent decrease in tissue oxygenation adversely affect wound healing in experimental animals subjected to these conditions, resulting in a slower gain of wound tensile strength.[28]

Diseases

Certain diseases lead to impaired wound healing. These are listed in Table 7-1.[29]

Systemic Medications[5,25,29,30,31,32,33]

Table 7-2 lists medications commonly incriminated as adversely affecting wound healing. Unfortunately, controlled clinical trials in humans are lacking.

Local Factors Affecting Wound Healing

Often, the clinician views healing as something that occurs after an injury has been sustained. It is important for us as dermatologic surgeons to remember that preoperative, intraoperative, and postoperative events affecting the healing site will ultimately determine its rate of healing, the efficacy of healing, and the avoidance of complications. I will briefly review the local factors that may play a role in wound healing.

Sterile Technique and Preparation of the Surgical Site

One of the more severe and unpredictable complications affecting dermatologic surgery is infection. Appropriate preparation before surgery of the surgeon and the surgical site is mandatory if infection is to be avoided.

A brief hand wash with soap under running water should be sufficient if the surgeon routinely gets into the habit of going through this ritual prior to beginning any new case. Highly effective surgical scrubs, such as Hibiclens (Stuart Pharmaceuticals—Wilmington, Delaware), are effective for most dermatologic surgical procedures. Indeed, studies have shown that the time-honored five-minute surgical scrub is not necessarily more effective than the brief scrub with an antiseptic detergent.[34,35]

Surgical gloves, either sterile or unsterile, are indicated today for all procedures in which the hands of the surgeon may be exposed to blood because of the risk of becom-

Table 7.1. Diseases Affecting Wound Healing[25]

A	B	C	D	E
Metabolic	Vascular	Hereditary	Immunologic Deficiencies	Other
1. Cushing syndrome	1. Atherosclerosis	1. Coagulation disorders	1. Chédiak-Steinbrinck-Higashi syndrome	1. Chronic pulmonary disease
2. Diabetes	2. Edema	2. Compliment deficiencies	2. Chronic granulomatous disease	2. Chronic liver disease
3. Fever	3. Heart failure	3. Ehlers-Danlos syndrome	3. G6PD deficiency	3. Malignancy
4. Hyperthyroidism	4. Hypertension	4. Prolidase deficiency	4. Job syndrome	
5. Malnutrition	5. Hypovolemia	5. Wermer's syndrome	5. Lazy leukocyte syndrome	
6. Renal failure	6. Vasculitis		6. Myeloperoxidase deficiency	
	7. Venous stasis		7. Sickle cell disease	

Table 7.2. Systemic Medications Affecting Wound Healing[5, 25, 29, 30, 31, 32, 33]

1. Accutane	11. Glucocorticoid
2. Anticoagulants	12. Local anesthetics
3. Antineoplastic agents	13. Metronidazole
4. Beta-amino propionitrile	14. Nicotine
5. Calcitonin	15. Nonsteroidal anti-inflammatory agents (NSAIDS)
6. Colchicine	
7. Cyclosporin A	16. Penicillamine
8. Dilantin	17. Salicylate
9. Epinephrine	18. Zinc sulfate
10. Ergotamine	

ing infected with hepatitis B or HIV.[36,37] While the incidence of transmission between patient and physician remains low, great caution must be exercised. Sterile gloves should be used in all cases of major incisional surgery. Surgical masks are necessary when large surgical incisions have been performed and when the procedure is a lengthy one, with the dermatologic surgeon talking over the wound in order to reassure the patient during the procedure.

Preparation of the surgical site before incision is aimed at removing as many transient and pathogenic bacteria as possible, and decreasing the resident bacterial flora of the skin to the lowest possible level. Keeping in mind that the skin cannot be completely sterilized, because 10–20% of the bacterial flora reside deeper within the pilosebaceous unit,[38] the surgeon should use the combined effects of a mechanical scrub with an effective antiseptic agent.[39] Gram-positive organisms tend to be the most common offending microbes for outpatient cutaneous surgery; gram-negative organisms affect wound infections in hospitalized patients much more than they would in surgery performed in the outpatient setting.

Hair removal at the surgical site before surgery should be performed only when hair will interfere with the surgery itself. Shaving causes cutaneous microinjury, and if it is to be done, it should be performed immediately before the surgery so that the chance of bacterial penetration and multiplication are kept to a minimum.[40,41,42] Table 7-3 lists some of the more common antiseptic agents used in dermatologic surgery, along with their advantages and disadvantages.

Intraoperative Events Affecting Wound Healing

Surgical technique is an important variable affecting the process of wound healing. Crushed and devitalized skin edges greatly increase the inflammatory reaction around the wound and promote secondary infection. As a result, gentle manipulation of tissue is mandatory during the procedure. Subcutaneous sutures should be neither too many nor too tight.[43] Wound closure, in regard to the cutaneous sutures, should similarly be under the least tension possible.

Hemostasis is also a critical part of skin surgery, which will have a significant impact on wound healing. In cases of large-vessel transection, suture ligature is preferable to abject electrocoagulation. Indeed, when one electrocoagulates, it is advisable to pick up the least amount of tissue with the hemostatic forceps so as to minimize unnec-

Table 7.3.   Antiseptic Agents in Dermatologic Surgery

Antiseptic Agent	Advantage	Disadvantage
Alcohol (isopropyl)	1. Inexpensive 2. Kills most bacteria 3. Effectiveness increases when combined with other antiseptics	1. Ineffective against spores 2. Slow antimicrobial action 3. Volatile 4. Corrosive to instruments 5. Irritating
Chlorhexidine (Hibiclens) 4% in sudsing base	1. Nonirritating 2. Covers gram-positive and gram-negative 3. Binds to stratum corneum 4. Does not get absorbed 5. Nontoxic 6. More prolonged suppression of bacterial growth 7. Cannot be removed by alcohol	1. Irritating to eyes and middle ear 2. Sudsing base very irritating
Hexachlorophene (Winthrop, New York, NY) (pHisoHex)	1. Good for gram-positive organisms	1. Bad for gram-negative organisms or fungi 2. Antibacterial film is removed easily with alcohol or soap 3. Easily absorbed through the skin 4. Causes neurotoxicity in infants 5. Teratogen
Hydrogen peroxide	1. Effective wound cleanser	1. No significant antiseptic properties
Iodoform (iodine plus polymer)	1. Good all around against gram-positive, gram-negative, and fungi	1. Skin reactions 2. Iodine toxicity in sensitive individuals 3. Do not leave a reliable residual of antibacterial activity

essary tissue damage. Other agents commonly used for hemostasis during dermatologic surgery include physical means such as pressure, which may control bleeding until more definitive measure can be taken, and cold, which by causing vasoconstriction allows time for coagulation to occur. However, cooling the skin to a temperature below 30° C may actually interfere with platelet aggregation, slow the coagulation cascade, and cause vasodilation thereafter. Bleeding times may then approach infinity when skin temperature approaches 0° C (32° F).[44] Bear in mind also that the chemical cauterants most commonly used by dermatologic surgeons cause significant tissue injury, which slows healing, and should not be used as hemostatic agents in wounds that will ultimately be sutured. Silver nitrate forms a thick eschar when silver ions combine with tissue protein to form insoluble precipitates, which occlude open vessels.[45] Monsel's solution (20% ferric subsulfate), because of its low pH and as a result of its subsulfate group, causes protein to denature and thus occlude blood vessels. Monsel's has a long-lasting cytotoxic effect.[46] Aluminum chloride's action is potentiated by its ability to hydrolyze to hydrochloric acid, which causes tissue coagulation and vasoconstriction. Because of this property, care must be taken when treating wounds around the eyes.

Notwithstanding the preceding considerations, inefficient hemostasis may lead to hematoma formation, with subsequent mechanical disruption of wound closure and the creation of conditions that favor the development of secondary infection. Indeed, meticulous but judicious hemostasis is critical to wound healing.

Infection is an important factor that may have a detrimental effect on wound healing. As complicating factors go, it is the most common local complication leading to prolonged healing.[47] Local tissue ischemia, foreign material within the wound, inappropriate preoperative precautions, and desiccation of tissue encourage the propagation of bacteria, which leads to a prolongation of the inflammatory phase of wound healing.[6] The cause in most instances is a gram-positive organism, but under unusual circumstances (eg, immunocompromised patients or diabetics) gram-negative organisms and *Candida albicans* may be implicated.[48]

The size and depth of the wound and whether it was allowed to heal by secondary intention or was repaired by primary closure, flap, or graft will obviously affect the duration of healing and the ultimate outcome and appearance of the cicatrix. We know that there are certain areas (predominantly concavities), especially on the face, that will tend to heal by secondary intention with minimal scarring. Furthermore, wound care and dressings should be modified to account for these differences. Tertiary intention (wounds that are surgically closed after the day of their creation) healing may necessitate antibiotic prophylaxis and more frequent dressing changes until appropriate granulation-tissue formation has been achieved and infection has been excluded.

BANDAGING/DRESSINGS

As dermatologic surgeons, it is natural for us to give great emphasis to the design as well as the mechanics of a particular procedure. On completion of that procedure, we frequently have the false impression that our entire task is completed and that some ethereal entity will now "mop up" and secure what we have so painstakingly accomplished. This entity frequently goes by the name of Judy or Manny or Jan, as it did for me during *my* training in dermatologic surgery. Through their great diligence, as well as the instruction that was transmitted to me by one of the authors of this text (HTG), it became crystal clear that bandaging spoke almost as highly (or detrimentally) of my work as did the actual surgery. Furthermore, postoperative follow-up and close supervision of my patients went a long way in establishing a trusting and compassionate physician–patient relationship, which made the provision of care less likely to be fraught with anxiety should an adverse event occur.

Bandaging is an art, after certain fundamentals are achieved, and therefore very few statements about dressing and bandaging should be dogmatic, because improvisation figures so prominently in their proper applications.

In this section, I will briefly discuss some of the basic principles of bandaging and dressings.

Purpose of Dressings

It is important to examine the purpose for dressings and to convey the principles involved in a simple fashion to our patients, or their families, after surgery has been performed.

1. *Absorption*, one of the primary functions provided by dressings, is dependent on the type of wound created, the depth of the wound, whether it was allowed to heal by secondary intention, and whether the integrity of the cutaneous surface was reconstructed by primary closure, flap, or graft. A general rule of thumb is that during the first phase of wound healing, there is significant exudate and transudate produced, and as a result, more frequent dressing changes will be necessary. As the inflammatory phase subsides and leads to the reconstructive phase, absorption becomes less important.

2. The second important function of dressings is to provide *pressure*, as this aids in hemostasis, in immobilizing skin edges, and ultimately in decreasing contraction. This does not mean that we should rely solely on dressings to achieve these goals; for proper hemostasis, good suturing technique and proper surgical design must be exercised before the application of the dressing.

3. Another important function that a dressing offers is *protection*. Trauma and contamination of the wound are the primary dangers, and as a result, the dressing should provide enough bulk to guard against these two events as much as possible.

4. Via *occlusion* the speed of reepithelialization increases under the proper dressing; it is thus important to convey this fact to the patient, who frequently has exactly the opposite view.

5. Another reason to continue using dressings until healing is achieved is the *psychological separation* of the wound from the patient and other family members. Undoubtedly, the patient is already experiencing significant stress as a result of having undergone the procedure. A proper dressing and good instructions given to the patient for care of the wound exhibit a sensitivity on the part of the physician that makes the patient feel that we, the surgeons, understand the stress that the procedure has caused and that we sympathize and are willing to aid the patient in preventing embarrassment that might be elicited in cases where the wound is left open.

Typical Dressing

Before the application of the dressing, make sure that there is no surgical debris on the wound. This can be achieved by cleansing the wound with hydrogen peroxide or saline. Hydrogen peroxide, which theoretically may interfere with wound healing, or sterile saline is especially helpful where clots, hair, or crusting are present. Before the dressing is applied, conduct a good visual inspection to rule out the possibility of oozing.

The typical dressing is made up of layers with specific functions. These are depicted in Table 7-4 and in Figures 7-1—7-6. As noted in Table 7-4, there are a variety of materials that can be used during bandaging, and individual cases require the analogous modification. Choice of the appropriate antibiotic ointment is a matter of preference, but make sure the patient has no previous history of sensitization to the substance to be used. The choice for contact and absorbent layers should be based on anatomic location, amount of anticipated oozing, and length of time from first application to first dressing change. The outer wrap layer has to be neat, because the patient will see it and as a result make a judgment as to the neatness and quality of the surgical work.

Table 7.4.   Wound Dressing Layers

Layer	Materials
A. Ointment	1. Polysporin
	2. Bacitracin
	3. Garamycin
	4. Bactroban
	5. Petrolatum
B. Contact Layer	1. Vaseline gauze
	2. Adaptic
	3. Aquaphor gauze
	4. Telfa
	5. Release
	6. N-Terface
	7. Vigilon
	8. Betadine gauze
	9. Xeroform, Xeroflo
	10. Op-Site, Tegaderm
C. Absorbent Layer	1. Cotton
	2. Dry gauze
	3. Eye pads
	4. Fluffed Kling
	5. Abd pads
	6. Dental rolls
D. Outer Wrap Layer	1. Paper tape
	2. Kling, Kerlix
	3. X-span
	4. Coban, Ace
	5. Hypafix

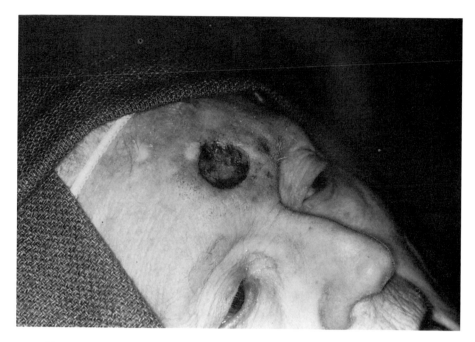

Figures 7.1–6.   Bandaging of forehead defect (Fig. 7-1) with a contact layer (Fig. 7-2); absorbent layers (Figs. 7-3 and 7-4) and outer wrap (Figs. 7-5 and 7-6). See Table 4.

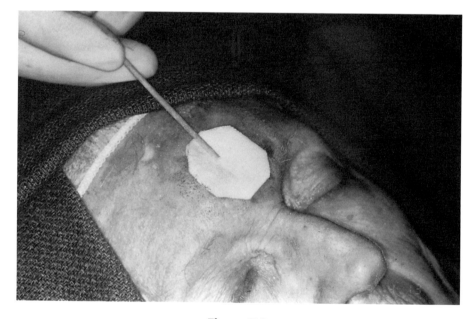

Figure 7.2.

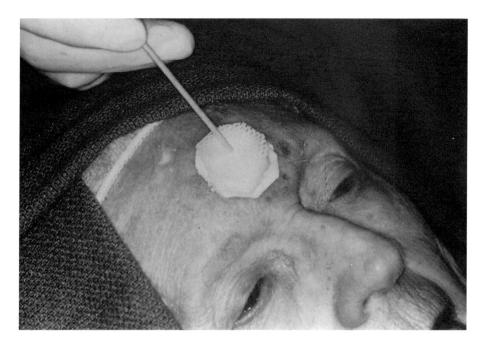

Figure 7.3.

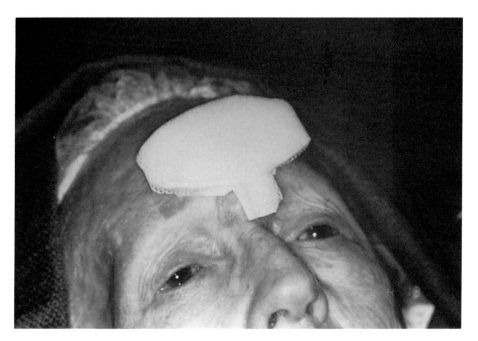

Figure 7.4.

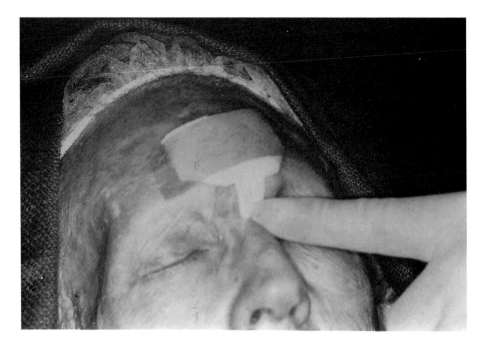

Figure 7.5.

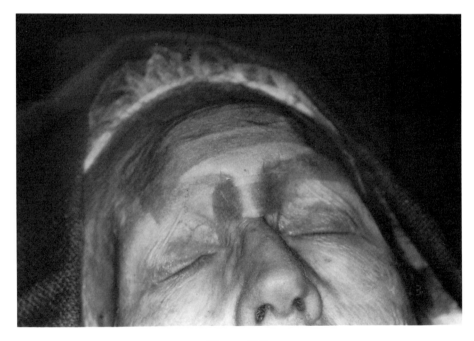

Figure 7.6.

In the case where a full-thickness or split-thickness skin graft is to be applied, a nonadherent contact layer substance has to be used. Adaptic gauze and N-Terface are two excellent examples. Telfa, although a good choice, may on occasion stick to the edges of a full-thickness or split-thickness skin graft, and care must be exercised when applying this material as the contact layer. In full-thickness skin grafts and split-thickness skin grafts, a bolster frequently has to be used. They are at times necessary for the facilitation of proper graft coaptation to the underlying wound bed, which is important during the first 48 hours after wounding. This usually can be made of cotton or an eye pad or sponge rubber and sutured into place. Sponge rubber bolsters, unless they are soaked in glycerin, should not be used directly over grafted skin because they will stick and make removal nearly impossible.

Occlusive and Biological Dressings

Until 1980, occlusive dressings were not readily available on the U.S. market. Today there are well over 30 occlusive dressings in use in the United States.[49] These have been used for the treatment of acute wounds to induce rapid epithelialization, reduce wound pain and tenderness, and produce a better cosmetic result.[50,51] In chronic wounds, the beneficial effect gained from occlusive dressings, as it pertains to debridement, far outweighs the risks of secondary infection.[50] Indeed, there may be a lower incidence of infection in acute and chronic wounds treated with occlusive dressings, probably owing to the relative impermeability of these dressings to exogenous bacteria and to neutrophils and other natural substances in the wound fluid that inhibit bacterial growth.[52,53]

To be most effective, occlusive dressings have to be placed on the wound shortly after surgery; maximum benefit as it pertains to re-epithelialization is achieved when these dressings are used within the first two hours after wounding.[54] The mechanism whereby occlusive dressings seem to speed epithelialization is related to their ability to effect growth-factor activities by keeping the wound fluid. The fluidity of the wound puts these growth factors in direct contact with healing tissue during the first 48 hours after wounding.[49]

Factors that may influence the use of occlusive dressings include availability, cost, instruction time, and the physician's knowledge of these materials. Table 7-5 outlines the four basic categories of occlusive dressings and their respective representatives. This list is being added to almost monthly, and newer and better dressings will continue to be developed. Generally, polyurethane films and hydrogels are used for acute wounds, and hydrocolloids and foams for more chronic wounds. It is important to note that occlusive dressings may, on occasion, convert a dry ulcer into a moist, exudating one, which may become difficult to manage for both physician and patient. During the 10–14 days that this conversion takes place, it may be necessary to change the dressing on an everyday or every-other-day basis. After this time, though, a single dressing may be worn for a week or more.

Biological Dressings

Porcine xenografts are the most widely used biological dressings. Their low cost, ease of storage, and low risk of acquired infection make them ideal for coverage of

Table 7.5. Occlusive Dressings

Films	Foams	Hydrocolloids	Hydrogels
TYPES	**TYPES**	**TYPES**	**TYPES**
OP-site	Synthaderm	Duoderm	Vigilon
Tegaderm	Epilock	Comfeel	Hydrogel
Bioclusive	LYO-foam A, C, T	Ulcer Dressing	Clear Site
Uniflex		Dermagran	Alginates
Oproflex	**CHARACTERISTICS**	Actiderm	Algiderm
Ensure-It			Sorbsan
Thin Film	Nonadherent,	**CHARACTERISTICS**	Algosteril
Blister Film	opaque		
Vari-moist	Polyurethane	Opaque	**CHARACTERISTICS**
Spray-ons	Moderate	Gas impermeable	
Omiderm	absorption	Very Absorbent	Absorbent
	For moderately	Separate from the	Nonadherent
CHARACTERISTICS	exuding wounds	wound as fluid	Semitransparent
		accumulates	
Polyurethane		Dressing should be	
Thin, transparent		changed only after	
Transmit h2O, O2, cO2		separation has	
Non absorbant		occurred	
		Thick discharge	

deeper wounds that are being allowed to heal by secondary intention or before a tertiary closure is to be performed.

Homografts (human cadaver skin) is an excellent product that is also used successfully while awaiting granulation to form beneath it. Cadaver skin, which has been irradiated and is safe from hepatitis B and HIV, can be used to cover large defects of the scalp. It can be left in place for periods ranging from one to two weeks.

Autografts (excess skin from a graft) can be placed in saline and frozen to be used at some later point. This is not often done because there are multiple other choices, as described previously.

Amniotic membranes have also been used in the past with mixed results, primarily over skin-graft donor sites.[55] For the practicing dermatologic surgeon, they are impractical, expensive, and cumbersome.

Dressings for Special Areas

Scalp

Large excisional wounds on the scalp and instances of hair transplantation and scalp reduction require the use of a full-head dressing. These are predominantly of two basic types, the turban type (Figure 7-7), whereby two Kling gauze rolls are used in interlocking fashion, or the modified Russian technique,[56] whereby the patient holds two ends of a 72–84 cm inch anchoring Kerlix gauze (width 7.6 or 10.2 cm) while another Kerlix roll is wrapped and intertwined perpendicularly to the anchoring roll in a turban fashion. The two vertical arms are subsequently secured under the chin.

Eyes

Extensive procedures involving the eyelids and the conjunctivae probably will require patching the eye so as to avoid corneal desiccation (Figure 7-8). Before patching the eye, a sterile ophthalmic antibiotic ointment (eg, Polysporin or Garamycin) should be applied. The eye is then closed and an eye pad is placed over it and secured tightly. This pad should be changed every 24 hours unless a full-thickness skin graft repair has been performed, in which case an oral antibiotic should be used and the dressing changed in five to seven days. If patching of a patient's eye is performed, that patient must be accompanied to and from the office and should not drive.

Nose

The greatest difficulty in applying a dressing to the nose usually involves situations where very large defects have been created or where there is the presence of exposed cartilage, either with perichondrium or stripped of it. Larger defects essentially require larger dressings, with care to secure the outer wrap layer with Mastisol (tincture of benzoin). Packing the nostril with a dental roll frequently helps in providing counterpressure in situations where a flap has been performed on the ala. Where the perichondrium has been stripped, great care must be taken not to allow the cartilage to become desiccated. This can be achieved by using a 2-mm trephine to punch out areas on the involved cartilage randomly, or by taking exceptional care, increasing the frequency of use of topical antibiotic ointment, and occluding this area over a large period

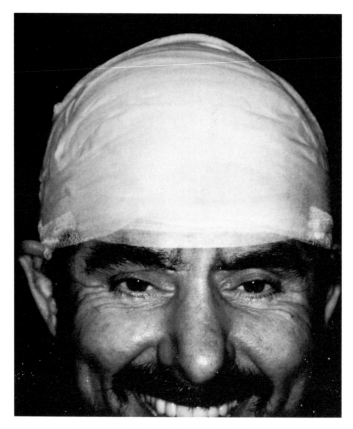

Figure 7.7. Turban type of scalp dressing for large wounds, hair transplantation or scalp reduction, or other procedures requiring a full head dressing.

of time to allow for granulation-tissue formation. In very large defects, where a large surface area of cartilage is exposed and where a repair is not possible, punching holes in the cartilage may be the only alternative.

Ear

The ear is the most common area to hemorrhage postoperatively. As a result, before dressing application, meticulous hemostasis must be attained. After this has been accomplished, it is important to provide the necessary bulk to the involved area and to secure the covering layer tightly with Mastisol. Packing the ear, both anteriorly and posteriorly and in the posterior auricular sulcus, also aids in the support of a potential full-thickness skin graft involving the scaphoid fossa or conchal bowl/external meatal os area (Figures 7-9 and 7-10). Wick-type dressings are frequently used after the first stage of an interpolation flap to repair a helical rim defect. These wick dressings are usually made of Xeroform (petrolatum) gauze dressings with additional antibiotic ointment wrapped around one or two dental rolls. These can be left in place for two to

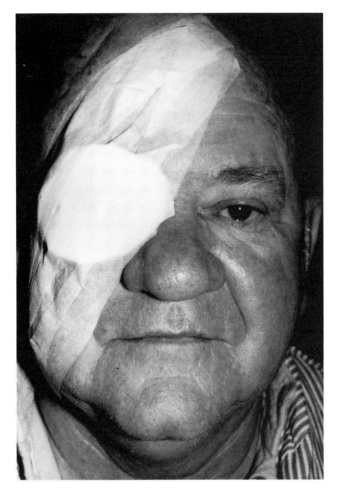

Figure 7.8. Eye patched with eye in closed position (upper lid covering cornea). Tape extends beyond bony prominences of zygoma and well onto forehead.

three days at a time and gently eased out with infiltration of sterile water or normal saline. Extreme care must be taken when cartilage is exposed here as well, because desiccation and secondary infection are a great likelihood. In borderline diabetics, or immunocompromised patients, it is advisable to use Bactroban ointment and cover with the appropriate antibiotic to prevent superinfection with *Pseudomonas*.

Lip

Because of a number of factors including mobility, the lip may be extremely difficult to bandage securely (Figures 7-11, 7-12, and 7-13). The patient may also be required to limit talking and eating (eg, the use of a soft diet may be in order).

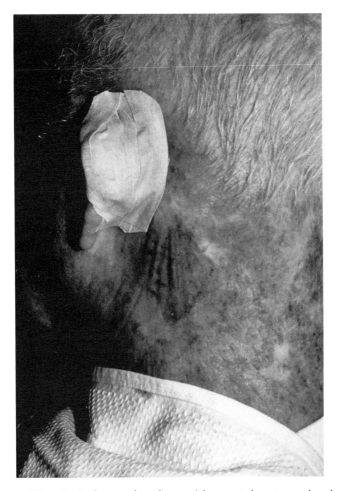

Figure 7.9.   Posterior ear bandage with care taken to pack sulcus.

Extremities

Procedures that lead to large wounds of the proximal upper and lower extremities need to be wrapped (Figure 7-14) with Coban or Kerlix gauze to completely immobilize the sutured area. The large underlying muscles exert shearing forces on the wound that may lead to wound separation, prolonged healing, and an unsightly scar. Wounds of the distal upper and lower extremities also must be immobilized; at times, especially for wounds that have been repaired by full-thickness skin graft or flaps involving the hands and feet, splints and possibly casts of these areas must be applied.

Dressings and splints of the distal upper and lower extremities must be applied with pressure, yet not strangulate circulation to the digits or toes. As a result, persistent pain or loss of acral sensation may be an indication to remove the dressing and reapply it in a looser fashion.

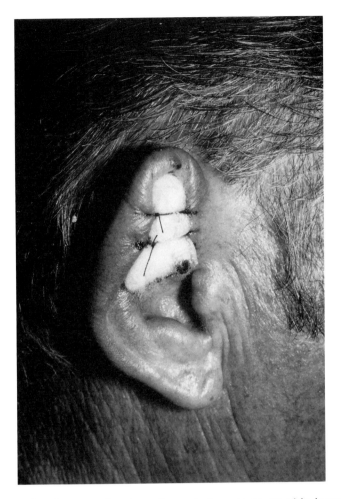

Figure 7.10. Sewn-on bandage for anterior ear to provide hemostasis and bolster-type bandage for underlying skin graft reconstruction.

POSTOPERATIVE INSTRUCTIONS

Dressing Removal

During the first 24 hours following a dermatologic surgical procedure, it is important for the patient to have the ability to get in contact with the dermatologic surgeon quickly in case an emergency should arise. It is my opinion that the first dressing change should be performed by the dermatologic surgeon or a member of the staff and that after this initial 24 hours, the patient may receive written instructions on wound care. Exceptions to this rule are permitted depending on the type of wound, its location, and the relative ability of the patient to manage the wound.

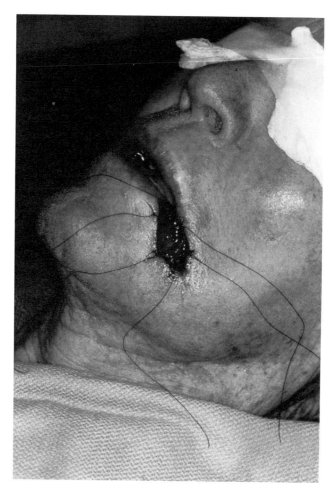

Figures 7.11, 7.12, 7.13.   Lower lip and commissure defect following Mohs surgery removal of extensive squamous cell carcinoma. Patient was then returned to referring physician for reconstruction to be done the following day. Overnight bandage followed the "layered principle" seen in Figures 1–6 with the use of a dental roll for bulk, pressure, and absorbency and with sutures used for security. Tape dressing at edge of mouth was coated with an ointment for protection against moisture.

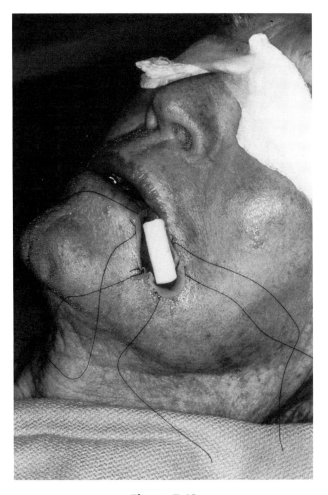

Figure 7.12.

When the initial dressing is removed, care must be taken to lift the contact layer gently and parallel to the incision. Perpendicular removal may result in pulling the sutures out and thus reopening the wound.

Postoperative pain medications and antibiotics should be used according to whether there is an indication and should be left to the judgment of the physician, depending on patient need and the clinical situation.

Showering or bathing are permitted depending on the type of procedure and the location of the procedure. It should be mentioned to the patient that he or she should shower or bathe with the dressing left in place; care of the wound should take place only after the bath is finished. I encourage the use of hydrogen peroxide as I feel it enables crust to loosen and thus not to adhere to the wound, thereby facilitating reepithelialization. Drying the peroxide and subsequently placing a thin film of antibiotic ointment with a nonadherent type of dressing rounds out the simple wound-care

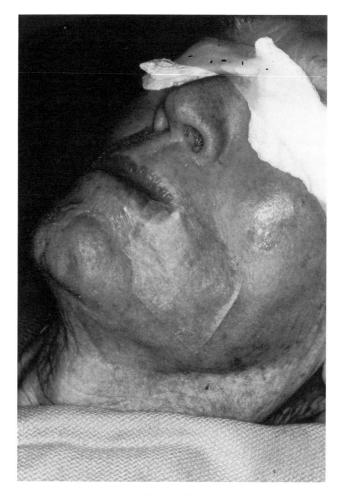

Figure 7.13.

instructions given to the patient. The patient is advised not to bend abruptly, not to lift heavy objects, and to avoid strenuous physical activity for approximately two weeks after the procedure.

CONCLUSION

This chapter has made an attempt at presenting some of the practical aspects of wound healing and bandaging. Experience in these two issues is gained through hands-on management of wound-care problems, imagination, ingenuity, and cooperation between physicians and nursing staff. It is important to remember that the phases of wound healing, location of the wound, and type of procedure performed ultimately determine the type and extent of bandaging that is required.

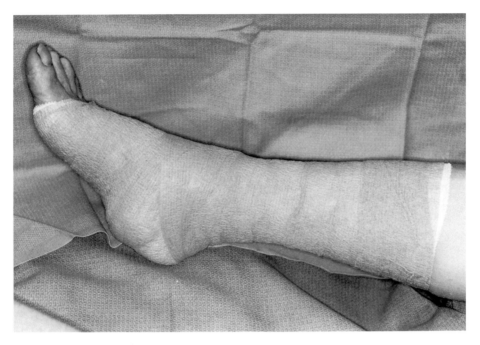

Figure 7.14. Wrapping of the extremity (again following the "layered principle") may be indicated in extremity wounds.

REFERENCES

1. Lyons AS, Petrucelli RJ. *Medicine, An Illustrated History.* New York, NY: Abradale Press; 1987:163.
2. Breasted JH. *The Edwin Smith Surgical Papyrus.* Vol. 1. Chicago, IL: University of Chicago Press; 1930.
3. Gamgee JS. Absorbent and medicated surgical dressings. *Lancet.* 1:127, 1880.
4. Bennett RG. *Fundamentals of Cutaneous Surgery.* St Louis, MO: CV Mosby; 1988:370.
5. Goslen JB. Wound healing for the dermatologic surgeon. *Dermatol Surg Oncol.* 14(9):959, 1988.
6. Clark, RAF. Cutaneous tissue repair: Basic biologic considerations. *I J Am Acad Dermatol.* 13:701, 1985.
7. Simpson DM, Ross R. The neutrophilic leukocyte in wound repair: A study with antineutrophil serum. *J Clin Invest.* 51:2009–2023, 1972.
8. Diegelmann RF, Choen IK, Kaplan AM. The role of macrophages in wound repair: A review. *Plast Reconstr Surg.* 68:107–113, 1981.
9. Winter GD. Formation of the scab and the rate of epithelialization of superficial wounds in the skin of the young domestic pig. *Nature.* 193:293–294, 1962.
10. Mayno G. The story of the myofibroblasts. *Am J Surg Path.* 3:535–542, 1979.
11. Kurkinen M, et al. Sequential appearance of fibronectin and collagen in experimental granulation tissue. *Lab Invest.* 43:47–51, 1980.
12. Balazs A, Holmgren HJ. The basic dye-uptake and the presence of growth inhibiting substances in the healing tissue of skin wounds. *Exp Cell Res.* 1:206–216, 1950.

13. Bentley JP. Rate of chondroitin sulfate formation in wound healing. *Ann Surg.* 165:186–191, 1967.

14. Wood GC. The formation of fibrils from collagen solutions: Effect of chondroitin sulfate and other naturally occurring polyanions on the rate of formation. *Biochem J.* 75:605–612, 1960.

15. Lark MW, et al. Close and focal contact adhesions of fibroblasts to a fibronectin-containing matrix. *Fed Proc.* 44:394–403, 1985.

16. Levenson SM, et al. The healing of rat skin wounds. *Ann Surg.* 161:293–308, 1965.

17. McGrath MH, Hundahl SA. The spatial and temporal quantification of myofibroblasts. *Plast Reconstr Surg.* 69:975–983, 1982.

18. Singer II, et al. In vivo co-distribution of fibronectin and actin fibers in granulation tissue: Immunofluorescence and electron microscope studies of the fibronexus at the myofibroblast surface. *J Cell Biol.* 98:2091–2106, 1984.

19. Zitelli JA. Wound healing and wound dressings. In: Roenigk RK, Roenigk HH (eds). *Dermatologic Surgery Principles and Practice.* New York, NY: Marcel-Dekker; 1989:97.

20. Knighton DR, et al. Regulation of wound healing angiogenesis: Effect of oxygen gradients and inspired oxygen concentration. *Surgery.* 90:262–269, 1981.

21. Knighton DR, et al. Oxygen tension regulates the expression of angiogenesis factor by macrophages. *Science.* 221:1283–1285, 1983.

22. Rheinwald JR, Green M. Serial cultivation of strains of human epidermal keratinocytes: The formation of keratinizing colonies from single cells. *Cell.* 6:331–344, 1975.

23. Barrandon Y, Green H. Three clonal types of keratinocytes with different capacities for multiplication. *Proc Natl Acad Sci USA 1987.* 84:2302–2306, 1987.

24. Phillips TJ. Wound healing and aging: An overview. *J Ger Derm.* 1(2):85–89, 1993.

25. Reed BB, Clark RAF. Cutaneous tissue repair: Practical implications of current knowledge II. *J Am Acad Dermatol.* 13:919–941, 1985.

26. Pollak SV. Wound healing: A review. III: Nutritional factors affecting wound healing. *J Dermatol Surg Oncol.* 5:615–619, 1979.

27. Hunt TK. Vitamin A and wound healing. *J Am Acad Dermatol.* 15:817–821, 1986.

28. Niinikoshi J. Effect of oxygen supply on wound healing and formation of experimental granulation tissue. *Acta Physiol Scand.* 78(Suppl 334):6–72, 1969.

29. Salmela K. Comparison of the effects of methylprednisolone and hydrocortisone on granulation tissue. *Scand J Plast Reconstr Surg.* 15:87–91, 1981.

30. Pollack SV. Systemic medications and wound healing. *Int J Dermatol.* 21:489–496, 1982.

31. Nemlander A, et al. Effects of cyclosporine on wound healing. *Transplantation.* 36:1–6, 1983.

32. Donoff RB. The effect of diphenylhydantoin on open wound healing in guinea pigs. *J Surg Res.* 24:41–44, 1978.

33. Boyce ST, Ham RG. Calcium-regulated differentiation of normal human epidermal keratinocytes in chemically defined clonal culture and serum free serial culture. *J Invest Dermatol.* 81:33–40, 1983.

34. Galle PC, et al. Reassessment of the surgical scrub. *Surg Gynecol Obstet.* 147:215–218, 1978.

35. Decher LA, et al. A rapid method for the presurgical cleaning of the hands. *Obstet Gynecol.* 51:115–117, 1978.

36. CDC. Recommendations for prevention of HIV transmission in health care settings. *MMWR.* 36:1–18, 1987.

37. Berberian BJ, Burnett JW. The potential role of common dermatologic practice technics in transmitting disease. *J Am Acad Dermatol.* 15:1057–1058, 1986.

38. Selwyn S, Ellis H. Skin bacteria and skin disinfection reconsidered. *Br Med J.* 1:136–140, 1972.

39. Maibach HI, Aly R. Sterilization and disinfection, in Epstein E, Epstein E, eds. *Skin Surgery,* 5th ed. Sprinfield, Ill: Charles C. Thomas; 1982:40–53.

40. Cruse PJE, Foord R. The epidemiology of wound infection: A ten year prospective study of 62,939 wounds. *Surg Clin North Am.* 60:27–40, 1980.
41. Seropian R, Reynolds BM. Wound infections after preoperative depilatory versus razor preparation. *Am J Surg.* 121:251–254, 1971.
42. Strachan C. Antibiotic prophylaxis in "clean" surgical procedures. *World J Surg.* 6:273–280, 1972.
43. Millewski PJ, Thomas H. Is a fat stitch necessary? *Br J Surg.* 67:393–394, 1980.
44. Larson PO. Topical hemostatic agents for dermatologic surgery. *J Dermatol Surg Oncol.* 14(6):623–632, 1988.
45. Helmkamp BF, et al. Effectiveness of topical hemostatic agents. *Contemp Obstet Gynecol.* 4:171–180, 1985.
46. Amazon K, et al. Ferrugination caused by Monsel's solution. *Am J Dermatopathol.* 2:197–205, 1980.
47. Silver IA. Cellular microenvironment in healing and non-healing wounds, in Hunt TK et al, eds. *Soft and Hard Tissue Repair.* New York, NY: Praeger Publishers; 1984:50–66.
48. Zitelli J. Wound healing for the clinician. *Adv Dermatol.* 2:243–268, 1987.
49. Eaglestein WH. Occlusive dressings. *J Dermatol Surg Oncol.* 19:716–720, 1993.
50. Falanga V. Occlusive wound dressings. *Arch Dermatol.* 124:872–877, 1988.
51. Hutchinson JJ. Prevalence of wound infection under occlusive dressings: A collective survey of reported research. *Wounds.* 1:123–33, 1989.
52. Mertz PM, et al. Occlusive wound dressings to prevent bacterial invasion and wound infection. *J Am Acad Dermatol.* 12:662–668, 1985.
53. Buchan IA, et al. Clinical and laboratory investigation of the compositions and properties of human skin wound exudate under semi-permeable dressings. *Burns.* 7:326–334, 1981.
54. Eaglestein WH, et al. Optimal use of an occlusive dressing to enhance healing. *Arch Dermatol.* 124:393–395, 1988.
55. Unger MG, Roberts M. Lyophilized amniotic membranes on graft donor sites. *Br J Plast Surg.* 29:99–101, 1976.
56. Lebovits PE, Dzubow, LM. A pressure dressing on the scalp by a modified Russian technique. *J Dermatol Surg Oncol.* 6:259–263, 1980.

8

POSTOPERATIVE CARE BEYOND THE BANDAGE TIME

Dudley Hill, FACD

INTRODUCTION

It is not always appreciated that wound healing continues for some months after injury. In the period following suture removal, appropriate wound care should enable the best possible results from skin surgery. This chapter deals with the subject of postoperative care beyond the bandage time.

WOUND HEALING

Cutaneous wound healing has been defined as the interaction of a series of phenomena that result in the resurfacing, reconstitution, and proportionate restoration of the tensile strength of the wounded skin.[1]

The dermatological surgeon must appreciate that wound remodeling continues over many months, and tensile strength takes time to develop (Figure 8-1); eg, after two weeks the scar is still fragile and has regained only 10% of its original strength. It follows that some wound support and reduced activity of the affected part is indicated during this time to allow the best wound healing.[2]

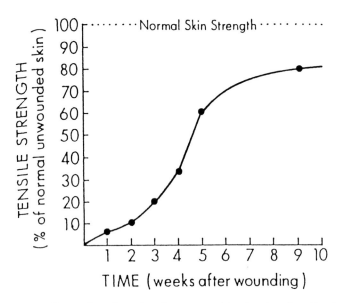

Figure 8.1.   Time taken for a healing wound to develop tensile strength.

IMMOBILIZATION

Patients are given routine instructions concerning care of the wound during the immediate postoperative period. These instructions should include appropriate immobilization of the affected part. It takes six to eight weeks for a wound to acquire final tensile
strength. To minimize the possibility of a stretch scar or dehiscence, advice concerning
immobilization must also be given following removal of the sutures.[3] Several factors
need to be considered in giving such advice:

1. the age of the patient
2. the preoperative level of physical activity
3. the site of the wound
4. the extent and depth of the wound

Many patients feel that a cutaneous surgical procedure is a minor event that will
temporarily interrupt their daily lives only for the time taken for the operation. They
need to be advised preoperatively about rest, immobilization, and reduction in their
normal physical activities in the postoperative period.

Wounds that have apparently healed normally and satisfactorily will sometimes
dehisce after suture removal simply because the patient has placed undue tension
across the wound by some physical exertion or movement. It is therefore most important to give firm and specific instructions preoperatively and to reinforce these instructions at the time of suture removal about what physical activities and movements
should be avoided and for how long.[3]

Advice about limitation of a patient's physical activity postoperatively is also
important in scheduling an appropriate time for a dermatological surgical procedure.

Many dermatological surgery procedures are not urgent; timing the procedure so that the patient can organize his or her activities appropriately will help to obtain the best results.

Areas where particular problems may arise are on the hand, wrist, and lower leg. Immediate postoperative rest and support using a sling and crepe bandage are often useful when operating on the hand and wrist. With large wounds there will always be some postoperative edema of the dorsum of the hand and the fingers. Although rest and elevation are helpful, dermatological surgeons must always be mindful of the need to maintain normal muscle activity and function, particularly in the small muscles of the fingers and the flexors and extensors around the wrist joint. The hand and wrist are the most used parts of the body in everyday living. It is necessary for dermatological surgeons to remember this when operating in those areas and to give specific instructions regarding remobilization and the extent of use allowable after suture removal.

Cutaneous wounds on the lower leg heal more slowly and can give more trouble than anywhere else on the body if the dermatological surgeon is not fully aware of potential problems. Preoperative advice about rest and elevation of the leg in the postoperative period is most important; the patient must be prepared so that the requisite time off and extra help at home, if necessary, can be organised. Sutures will seldom be removed in less than 14 days and may be left in for up to 21 days in some circumstances. The lower leg is an area where the cutaneous blood supply is not the best even in young, healthy individuals. Hence the need for rest and elevation postoperatively, the duration of which will depend on the extent of the wound, the age of the patient, and the blood supply to the area. Patients who have symptoms or signs of peripheral vascular disease or venous hypertension, or who are diabetic or chronic smokers must be told that they are particularly at risk for poor healing or dehiscent wounds on the lower leg following surgery.[3] In such patients consideration may be given to a period of rest and leg elevation in hospital in the immediate postoperative period. Gradual reintroduction of activity should be advised. A lower-leg–supporting stocking is often useful after suture removal and may be worn during the day for several months. Resumption of normal walking and running activities may begin six to eight weeks postoperatively.

Finally, instructions concerning immobilization need to be individualized. Increasing movement and exercise should be phased in during regular review of the healing wound. The patient needs to understand the reasons for the immobilization. Common sense and the factors discussed previously should allow appropriate advice for each individual and his or her wound.

WOUND SUPPORT

Once the sutures are removed from a wound it is advisable to provide further support to the healing scar to provide the best possible cosmetic results. As stated previously, wounds possess only 10% of their tensile strength at about two weeks. If any wound is under any stress or tension, it follows that the scar is likely to either 1) dehisce, 2) develop a spread scar, or 3) develop a hypertrophic scar. The support provided depends on the area involved and the extent of the wound. Certain areas are prone to develop hypertrophic or spread scars—notably the upper trunk, shoulders, upper arms, and thighs.[4,5] In these areas it is always advisable to use slowly absorbable sutures to close the subcutaneous space and allow the epidermis to be opposed without tension.[6,7] Polyglycolic acid (Dexon), polydioxane sulfate (PDS), or polyglactin 910 (Vicryl) sutures are currently favored and are used in this area as buried sutures. In other areas, closure of the subcutaneous space and opposition of epidermal edges in everted fashion without tension is also advisable to achieve the best results. In areas where the wound is either superficial or under no tension (eg, the eyelids) deeper sutures may not be necessary.

Once nonabsorbable sutures are removed from a wound, additional support while the wound gains strength is advised.[8] This can be achieved by using adhesive tapes (such as steristrips or micropore paper tape) or the more elegant stretch adhesive tapes (eg, Hypafix, Fixomull, or Mefix). Ideally, such support should continue for two to four weeks postoperatively. This requires good patient compliance. Patient cooperation is more likely if the reason for the use of the supporting tape is explained. Daily reapplication of the support tape is preferred, although some patients like to leave the stretch-type adhesive tapes in place for two or three days at a time. Some patients do not like the appearance of these supporting tapes on the face for weeks at a time; in such cases, a compromise application of the supporting tapes overnight only is still useful. The tape should be applied first on one side of the wound and then stretched over the scar to adhere to the other side (Figures 8-2, 8-3, and 8-4). Occasional allergic or irritant reactions to the adhesive occur,[3] so patients must be warned to advise of any such reaction.

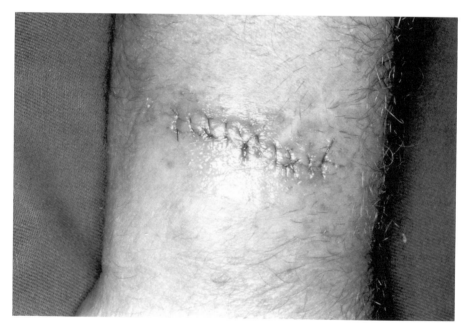

Figure 8.2.   Healing wound on dorsum of wrist before suture removal at 12 days.

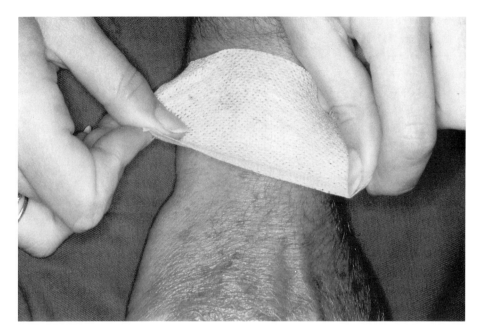

Figure 8.3.   Fixomull stretch adhesive dressing applied on one side of the wound, then stretched before application on the other side to provide support.

SKIN GRAFTS

Skin grafts are not uncommonly used to repair defects in dermatological surgery. Split-thickness skin grafts are used for larger defects; full-thickness skin grafts are used for smaller defects on the face, particularly on the nose, eyelids, and ears. Good preoperative counseling about the graft's appearance during the first few weeks will alleviate many of the patient's concerns.[9]

Both split-thickness and full-thickness grafts require initial immobilization and some form of pressure dressing to keep the graft adherent to the base of the wound. Once the pressure dressing is removed the graft will appear depressed. Grafts are often multicolored and crusted at the time of suture- and pressure-dressing removal. Patients should be informed about the likely appearance of the graft at this stage and reassured that it is normal.

The patient also needs to be advised that the final result following a skin graft will be apparent only after several weeks or months. They need to know that subcutaneous tissue regeneration will fill the graft out over a four- to six-week period. The graft is still fragile after initial dressing removal and should have a light, protective dressing for the subsequent week. Even after the graft has become uniformly colored and healed, the surface is often scaly and dry, and the borders of the graft may often be felt as a palpable ridge of scar tissue. The application of a simple moisturizer such as petroleum jelly,[10] with regular massage to the graft margins, will improve the appearance of the graft and enable the patient to feel that he or she is contributing to the final result. If a

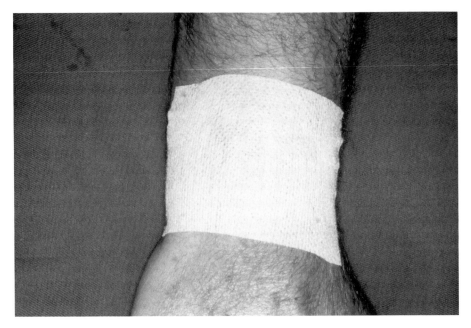

Figure 8.4. Fixomull stretch adhesive dressing in place.

graft does not give a satisfactory result, consideration may be given to localized dermabrasion[11] at about eight weeks. If this possibility is discussed preoperatively, or at the time of surgery, then the patient's acceptance will be much greater.

MOISTURIZERS

Moisturizers are cosmetic products developed and marketed for the treatment and relief of dry skin. Dry skin is a well-known side effect of chronic sun damage. People living in climates with low humidity will also be particularly prone to dry skin. The use of regular moisturizers returns moisture and hydration to the skin and is therefore active both as a treatment and as a prophylactic.

Moisturizers constitute a broad category including creams, lotions, and bath oils. In the United States moisturizers are one of the fastest-growing segments of the cosmetic industry. This may be because the advertising message to the consumer is that dry skin is aging skin. Moist skin is equated with beautiful and youthful skin whereas dry skin is shown as a sign of the aging process.

Moisturizing creams used to treat dry skin are divided into two types. The first type is oil in water, with water as the dominant component; the second type is water in oil, with the oil as the dominant and continuous phase. Water-in-oil products have a longer-lasting emollient or moisturizing effect. They are more commonly used as night creams, lubricating creams, or cold creams. Most people prefer less oily products; facial moisturizers and moisturizing creams marketed as hand lotions tend to be oil-in-water compounds. There has been an increasing trend lately toward the use of lotions as face and body moisturizers. Oil-in-water moisturizing lotions contain more water than the corresponding creams. Such moisturizing lotions are convenient to use and are becoming increasingly popular because of their higher water content.

Various compounds may be added to basic moisturizers to both enhance their effectiveness and provide a more cosmetically appealing product. Currently there is a trend to add various alpha hydroxy acids (fruit acids) to provide enhanced moisturization and a slight peeling effect that allows increased penetration of the moisturizer. In the low concentrations used in moisturizers these alpha hydroxy acids are nonirritating, but their use in higher concentrations in chemical peeling is irritating. Another compound that may be added is urea, which acts as a humectant and provides increasing moisturization to the skin with only a low concentration of urea.

Moisturizers are highly effective, clinically proven therapies and are safe for dry and sensitive skin, including aging skin. They are also effective when the skin is irritated by other agents that may promote drying, such as topical retinoic acid. There are a wide variety of moisturizers currently available, a number of which are promoted for special areas such as the face. Price is not always a good indicator of the effectiveness of moisturizing products. A number of studies have indicated that the simpler and less expensive formulations may be just as effective as the more complex, higher-priced products.

Moisturizers increase the water content of the skin, and their emollient action softens the skin. The use of moisturizers on a daily routine basis will help patients maintain a more healthy skin that looks and feels better.

In addition to aiding dry and sun-damaged skin, the regular use of moisturizers has been reported to allow more rapid healing and better cosmetic results following procedures such as dermabrasion and chemical peeling.[10]

SUN PROTECTION

Much dermatological surgery involves the treatment of skin cancer. General advice should therefore be given about sun protection of the skin and about the association between sun exposure and skin cancer. Although the majority of skin cancer sufferers are over 50 and have considerable preexisting sun damage, it is still important to advise them that sun protection will help reduce the rate at which any further skin cancers may develop. This advice has been given added credence following publication of an article entitled "Reduction of Solar Keratoses by Regular Sunscreen Use" in the *New England Journal of Medicine*.[12] This article is the first published proof that regular use of sunscreens is effective in humans both for preventing the development of solar keratoses and for hastening the remission of existing ones.

It is also worth advising patients of the association between sun exposure and photoaging of the skin. Many patients are unaware that the majority of changes they associate with chronological aging—irregular pigmentation, telangiectasia, wrinkling, and senile ecchymoses—are in fact mainly due to the chronic accumulated effects of sun exposure.

Sun-protection advice should include more than just the use of a sunscreen. In Australia, Anti-Cancer Councils and the Australasian College of Dermatologists have popularized the following catchy slogan

SLIP on a shirt
SLOP on a sunscreen
SLAP on a hat

to highlight the three major methods by which personal sun protection can be applied (Figure 8-5).

Slip on a shirt—a closely woven shirt, preferably with a collar and sleeves, is advised. A rough method of detecting how effective a particular shirt will be as a sunscreen involves holding a shirt up to the light to see how much it lets through. Slop on a sunscreen—with increasing public awareness about the association between skin cancer and sun exposure there has been an explosion (at least in Australia) in the use of sunscreens. Pharmaceutical companies have responded by manufacturing an increasing range of sunscreens. Australians are encouraged to use a broad spectrum sunscreen with an SPF factor of 15 or more. Modern sunscreens of this type usually contain two or more active chemicals that provide greater than 94% protection in the UVB range (290–320 nm) and greater than 90% protection in the lower UVA range (320–360 nm).[13] The inclusion of an inert reflective sunscreen material such as titanium dioxide in many broad-spectrum sunscreens in recent times has provided increased effectiveness across the entire ultraviolet spectrum. Other thick, inert-type reflective sunscreens incorporating zinc oxide remain popular on localized areas, such as the nose, that receive a high incidence of UV light.

Slap on a hat—a broad-brimmed hat with at least a 10-cm brim is necessary to give maximum protection for the neck and ears as well as the face. Wearing such a hat will

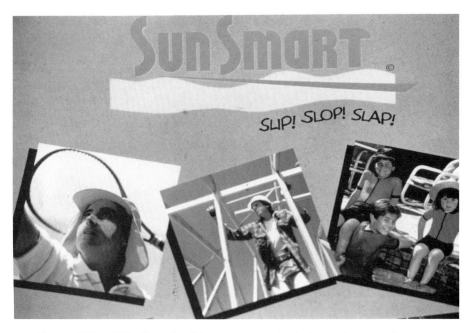

Figure 8.5.   "Slip Slop Slap" is now a standard phrase in Australian sun-protection literature.

provide about 70% protection to the face from incident UV light.[14] The protection provided decreases rapidly with smaller brim sizes (Figure 8-6).

In addition to "Slip Slop Slap," sun-protection advice should also include a) the fact that two thirds of the incident ultraviolet light during a day occurs between the hours of 10 AM to 2 PM (11 AM to 3 PM in those areas that have daylight saving in summertime), the hours when UV intensity is highest and when direct exposure should be avoided if possible; and b) the little-known fact that the UV intensity is not directly related to the ambient temperature. In Australia most weather bulletins on the major TV and radio stations now include information about the UV intensity as well as the day's temperature. Thus UV intensity may be extremely high on a comparatively cool day and may even be quite high on a day with considerable cloud cover. Sunburn occurring on such days has given rise to the myth of "windburn."

Anticancer councils and dermatology associations in most countries with a significant incidence of skin cancer have brochures detailing this information in an easy to read form (Figure 8-7). These brochures are most useful in disseminating appropriate information about sun protection and can be given preoperatively to patients along with other information sheets.

LONG TERM FOLLOW-UP

Skin Cancer Patients

Patients should be made aware that the development of a skin cancer means an increased chance of further skin cancers appearing. This applies to all forms of skin cancer.

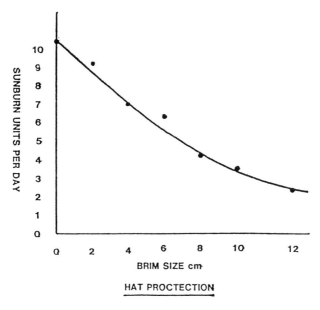

Figure 8.6.   Graph illustrating level of protection provided according to brim size of hat—by kind permission of Dr W. Ryman.

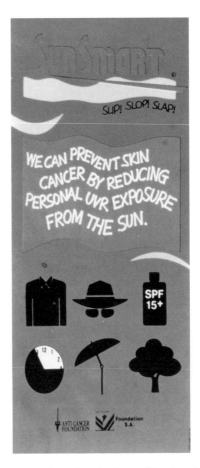

Figure 8.7.   The cover of a simple but effective brochure illustrating methods of sun protection.

A number of studies support the contention that patients with a first primary skin cancer are at a higher risk than nonaffected individuals of developing a further primary skin malignancy.[15,16] One study involving 6310 patients from Arizona[15] with a primary nonmelanoma skin cancer reported that those with a primary basal cell carcinoma had almost a 50% chance of developing a second primary tumor over a period of 3 1/2 years. For primary cutaneous squamous cell carcinomas the risk was lower at just under 20%. The risk of developing a second primary melanoma has been previously reported at between 3% and 6%.[17] Those patients who develop melanoma in a setting of multiple atypical moles have an even greater chance of developing a second melanoma.[18] There is also evidence from the Arizona study and others[19] that a patient with one type of skin cancer is at increased risk of developing other types of primary skin cancer. The results of these studies are sufficient evidence for regular review of skin cancer patients with the aim of detecting further primary skin cancers as early as possible. Fears concerning the future effects of a reduced ozone layer[20] and evidence of a continuing increase in the incidence of all forms of skin cancer[21,22] add further weight to the fact that regular follow-up for skin cancer sufferers should be mandatory.

Follow-up examinations for skin cancer patients may include total examination of the skin surface, review of any previously treated areas, and palpation of any relevant lymph nodes. Further investigations are usually only required in the presence of positive signs or symptoms.

Such follow-up examinations need not necessarily always be carried out by the treating dermatological surgeon. A competent family practitioner or dermatologist may be more appropriate. The treating dermatological surgeon, however, should explain that longer-term follow-up is necessary and at what intervals it is deemed appropriate. The timing of follow-up examinations needs to be individualized according to

a) the severity of associated sun damage
b) the past history of skin cancers—obviously a past history of multiple frequent skin cancers will require more frequent follow-up.
c) the type of skin cancers—a patient treated for a thick melanoma will need more frequent follow-up than one with a single BCC.
d) other factors, eg, patients on long-term immunosuppression (such as those with organ transplants) are at greater risk of developing frequent and aggressive skin cancers. Patients with the basal cell nevus syndrome or xeroderma pigmentosum will also develop frequent skin cancers. These patients need regular and frequent review at least every three months.

The Arizona study[15] suggested that patients treated for nonmelanoma skin cancers should be followed up every 3 months for the first 12 months, as this was the period with the highest incidence of second primary skin cancers. Thereafter, intervals of 6 to 12 months were advised for life.

Patients who have been treated for melanoma also need to be followed up long term. A three- to six-months' review is suggested for the first 24 months and thereafter less frequently. A proposed regimen for follow-up after excision of a primary cutaneous melanoma based on tumor thickness[23] would appear to be a logical approach. The recent observation that metastases from thin melanomas tend to appear late (up to five years or even longer from treatment of the primary melanoma) confirms the necessity for prolonged follow-up for all melanoma patients.

Patients with skin cancer also need to be given advice about the signs and symptoms of skin cancer. Understanding by the patient of the physical signs and presentation of basal and squamous cell carcinomas and the ABCD of melanoma will often allow skin cancers to be detected and treated at an early stage. Brochures produced by dermatology associations or anticancer councils are most useful in reinforcing this message. "A picture is worth a thousand words"; most of these brochures will show pictures of typical examples of skin cancers together with appropriate descriptions. Patients find such brochures useful and appreciate their dermatological surgeon's concern about their future well-being.

Non–Skin Cancer Patients

Patients operated on for reasons other than skin cancer need to be followed up until a "final result" has been achieved. This plan should be explained to the patient at the outset and will vary according to the procedure and the patient.[24]

Constant reassurance of patients that everything is progressing normally is helpful and allays anxiety, particularly with cosmetic procedures. Patients expect some dramatic changes in the immediate postoperative period—edema, bruising, erythema, crusting, and discomfort. Once these acute changes have settled, however, there is an intermediate period until the final result is achieved. Depending on the particular procedure this is often a comparatively slow change and is the time when patients need most reassurance and encouragement.

No set time for follow-up visits can be laid down. It is important, however, that the patient knows that the surgeon is interested in his or her particular case and that he is always available for consultation if the patient has any concerns. Realism combined with honest optimism concerning the final result is the best approach.

COMMON POSTOPERATIVE FINDINGS FOLLOWING SUTURE REMOVAL

Any surgical procedure will result in a risk of producing "problems" for the patient. This applies particularly to dermatological surgery because the changes are visible and obvious to the patient and his or her family, friends, and associates. An expected change is not a "problem," an unexpected change may become one.

Patients are generally not very knowledgeable about the changes associated with wound healing. The treating surgeon should therefore make the patient aware of the anticipated changes in and around the healing wound before the time of surgery. A little time spent explaining the expected changes and the anticipated outcome of cutaneous surgery before the procedure may save considerable time and effort in the postoperative phase. It is imperative that the expectations of patient and surgeon should coincide, regarding both short-term changes and long-term results.

Information sheets are useful allies but can never totally replace surgeons who have a caring attitude and show concern for the well-being of their patients both at the time of surgery and postoperatively. Fully informed patients will cause fewer problems for surgeons in the long run.

It is also appropriate to inform the patient that compliance with instructions regarding dressings, resting the affected part, reduced physical activity, and wound support is important if the best result is to be achieved. One can explain that the final result will be brought about by the combined efforts of the surgeon *and* the patient.[25]

Particular postoperative findings (as opposed to complications, which are covered in Chapter 9) that may occur and require explanation after suture removal or beyond the bandage time include the following:

a) edema
b) dysesthesia
c) telangiectasia
d) discomfort
e) appearance of the scar
f) reactions within the scar
g) contour imperfections
h) asymmetry
i) pigmentary changes

Edema

Swelling within and around surgical wounds is to be expected. This may be due to either a reaction to tissue injury or to lymphatic obstruction.

The acute edema following cutaneous surgery due to tissue injury normally settles down within a few days. The extent and duration of such edema depends on the amount of tissue injury during surgery. No specific treatment is usually required, although pressure dressings and cold packs[3] may help limit such edema to some degree. A special area that may cause concern for the patient is the periorbital edema in the loose tissue of the eyelids that almost invariably follows surgery to the forehead, temple, cheek, or periorbital area.

Edema secondary to lymphatic obstruction may be more long lasting. This may occur in some flaps with a narrow base when it may contribute to pincushioning or trap-door formation. Edema secondary to lymphatic obstruction may also be seen in the periorbital area, particularly the lower eyelid, following surgery to the zygomatic area.[26] Such lymphatic edema may take weeks or even months to resolve completely.

Surgery around the ankle and lower leg is also commonly followed by some persistent swelling of the foot and ankle that may continue for weeks or even months. The use of a below-the-knee support stocking during the day is useful in such cases. Similarly, persistent edema of the fingers following surgery of the hand is not uncommon, but should eventually disappear after being present for weeks to months. Rest and elevation of the arm in a sling will limit edema formation immediately following hand surgery. A program of gradually increasing movement of both wrist and fingers thereafter should prevent any residual joint stiffness and allow the wound to heal satisfactorily.

Dysesthesia

Loss of sensation, partial or complete, is not uncommon following cutaneous surgery. On the face, sensory nerves (which are branches of the trigeminal nerve) run in a comparatively superficial plane in many areas, and are often severed during skin cancer surgery. The resulting numbness or parasthesia will usually disappear over time. Resolution may take 6 to 12 months or sometimes even longer. The exact mechanism of sensory recovery is not clear, but patients can be reassured that complete recovery is almost invariable.

A particular area where sensory loss can be predicted postoperatively is in the upper forehead following horizontally placed incisions that sever branches of the supraorbital and supratrochlear nerves as they run vertically above the frontalis muscle. The resulting paresthesiae of the upper forehead and scalp superior to the wound are noticed particularly when brushing or combing the hair.

Skin grafts and some flaps will also show loss of sensation for several weeks or months. Once again, full recovery usually occurs.

Telangiectasia

Wounds that are under some tension will sometimes heal with the development of marked telangiectasia on either side of the scar. This may cause a cosmetic problem, particularly on the face. The nose seems to be particularly prone to develop this change (Figure 8-8), and there also appears to be an individual predisposition. This telangiec-

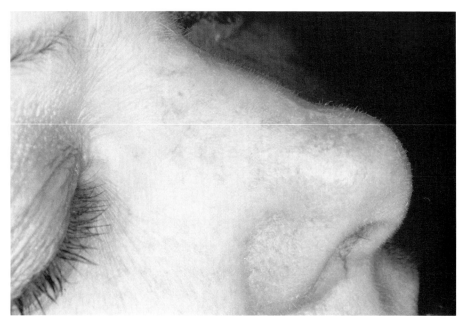

Figure 8.8. Telangiectasia on either side of a scar following a nasal flap repair.

tasia tends to be permanent. If it presents a problem appropriate laser treatment or sclerotherapy is usually successful.[27]

Discomfort

Most patients are agreeably surprised by the lack of discomfort or pain that follows cutaneous surgery. Severe pain in the immediate postoperative period may indicate an impending infection or developing hematoma. Pain or discomfort that persists after wound healing may have a number of causes:

(1) persistent perineural involvement by skin cancer. Typically such pain will start some weeks or even months after the initial wound has healed and tends to be episodic and shooting.[28]

(2) Healing scar tissue may entrap nerves, giving rise to pain or discomfort localized to the scar.

(3) Cut nerves may heal with the formation of traumatic neuromas, giving rise to pain that tends to occur on local pressure on or round the scar.

Appearance of the Scar

The dermatological surgeon should always aim for the best possible result. In most instances attention to scar placement, proper surgical techniques, and appropriate postoperative care will result in a soft, fine-line scar that is almost invisible.[29] In certain areas and with closure of some defects, however, such a perfect result is not always achievable, even with the best care. Where less than ideal scars are likely, the surgeon should warn the patient preoperatively of that possibility. As previously stated, the "cape" area of the upper trunk and shoulders is notorious for spread and hypertrophic scars, so patients should be warned accordingly.

Some patients have a particular predisposition to form hypertrophic scars. Such a history of previous scarring should be sought preoperatively. Postoperative use of pressure dressings[30] or silicone gel sheeting[31] and early intervention with intralesional steroid injections[5] may help reduce or prevent such scars in these patients.

Where a wound heals under some tension, spreading of the scar is almost inevitable.[32] Wound support for several weeks after surgery, immobilization in the immediate postoperative period, and reduced physical activity may help reduce the extent of scar spreading.

Nasal skin that has wide and patulous pilosebaceous openings tends to heal with depressed, slightly spread scarlines[29] no matter how careful the surgeon is (Figure 8-9).

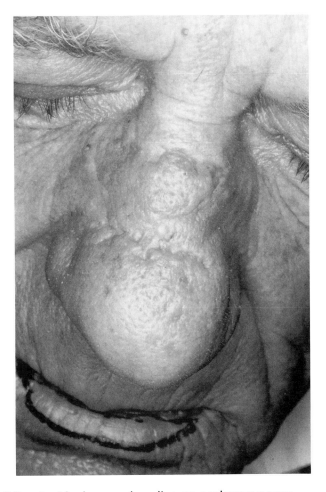

Figure 8.9.   A wide depressed scarline on a sebaceous nose.

Reactions in the Scar

A number of reactions appearing as cysts, nodules, plaques, or areas of inflammation may arise within a scar sometime after healing. These reactions are often a cause for concern, particularly if the surgery was for skin cancer.

The etiology of such reactions include

1) epidermoid inclusion cyst
2) foreign body reactions
3) spitting suture.

Epidermoid Cysts

These may appear weeks or even months postoperatively as small milial or larger epidermoid cysts. They may be due to cyst formation from epidermis that was buried at the time of surgery, transected pilosebaceous follicles, or epidermized suture tracks. Sometimes their appearance is associated with surrounding inflammation but more often they arise as small, asymptomatic papules or nodules within or immediately adjacent to the healed scar. In many cases simple incision with a sterile needle or scalpel blade and evacuation of the keratinous contents is all that is necessary to resolve them.

Foreign Body Reaction

Granulomatous inflammatory reactions may occur within or adjacent to a scar secondary to retained suture material or to other foreign material that may have been left in the wound such as cotton, talc from gloves, or hair.[33] Such reactions may arise days or weeks after healing. The causative foreign body may be spontaneously expelled, but sometimes a small incision may be necessary to remove the retained material.

Spitting Suture

Buried sutures are well known to extrude through the healed scar at times. This event is usually discovered some weeks after healing and most commonly has little or no associated inflammation. The retained sutures are usually easy to remove.

The absorbable suture in common use may remain in place for months although they lose their strength after several weeks. Spitting sutures are said to occur more often with polyglactic acid sutures or when the suture is placed more superficially. Tying the knot proximal to the skin surface rather than burying it deeply is also thought to increase the frequency of spitting sutures.

Contour Imperfections

Repair of facial defects by flaps or grafts may result in some changes in local skin contours. It must be remembered that the remodeling phase of wound healing is slowly progressive and continues for many months postoperatively. This remodeling will usually correct the majority of minor contour imperfections. Reassurance and encouragement of the patient in these cases is usually all that is required.

In some instances, such as localized trap-door or pincushion deformities, intralesional steroid injections given every three to six weeks will hasten resolution.

The nose is an area where contour deformities are particularly noticeable. When nasal contour changes are a problem, local dermabrasion can be useful to correct such changes. It is always worthwhile preparing the patient for a two-stage procedure when repairing nasal defects.

Skin grafts will often result in some localized contour change. Providing the patient is prepared for the long period over which grafts mature, and is advised about the eventual likely result, there are usually no problems. Intralesional steroids to hypertrophic areas, scar revision,[34] and dermabrasion[35] may all help improve any contour imperfections in skin grafts.

Asymmetry

When large defects on the face are repaired, particularly if local flaps are used, some postoperative asymmetry of facial features is not uncommon. Providing the flap is well planned, this asymmetry should correct itself. Thus, an eyebrow may be lifted up to 10 mm postoperatively but will usually return to its normal position after several weeks.[36] A somewhat smaller upward pull is allowable on the upper lip, but this too will usually fall back into its original position with time.

Dermatological surgeons must be particularly aware of asymmetrical changes induced in the nostrils and nasal ala area.[37] Asymmetry in this area is a cause for considerable concern in many patients and tends to be quite noticeable. Dorsal nasal and other flaps on one side of the nose will usually result in some initial asymmetry. Providing this is minor, it will correct itself in time.

Asymmetry in some areas is quite acceptable. For example, providing the curvature of the helical rim is maintained, most patients are not concerned if one ear is markedly smaller than the other. Likewise, some loss of the lateral eyebrow is usually not a problem, whereas even a small loss of the medial eyebrow causes considerable comment.

It is most important, either before or at the time of surgery, that patients be advised about any anticipated changes in facial symmetry. Reassurance that these changes will correct themselves will allow the patient to accept them and not cause him or her any postoperative problems.

Pigmentary Changes

In white patients most scars become hypopigmented with time. This is particularly evident after electrodessication or cryotherapy. A well-healed excision scar also becomes hypopigmented in time. In patients with plethoric facial skin, these hypopigmented scars will show up a little more than in people with paler skin.

Hyperpigmentation of scars is less common but may be seen in certain circumstances. People with darker skin may develop hyperpigmentation, although this is usually found in the skin around the scar and is a result of postinflammatory changes. This should eventually resolve spontaneously. Excessive use of ferric subsulfate solution (Monsel's solution) for hemostasis has been reported to produce scar pigmentation.

SUMMARY

Care of healing wounds after suture removal has not received a great deal of attention in the dermatological surgery literature. This postoperative period is, however, important if best final results from cutaneous surgery are to be achieved. This chapter outlines the various factors that must be considered during this time and the various ways to help the healing wound and the patient achieve the best possible outcome. Particular emphasis is placed on attempting to anticipate possible problems and in keeping the patient fully informed.

Finally, the importance of being available to help with any problems the patient might have during the postoperative period and presenting a caring and reassuring attitude cannot be overemphasized.

REFERENCES

1. Goslen JB. Wound healing for the dermatologic surgeon. *J Dermatol Surg Oncol.* 14:9, 959–972, 1988.
2. Hardy MA. The biology of scar formation. *Phys Ther.* 69:1014–1024, 1989.
3. Telfer NR, Moy RL. Wound care after office procedures. *J Dermatol Surg Oncol.* 19:722–731, 1993.
4. Murray JC, Pollack SV, Pinneic SR. Keloids: A review. *J Am Acad Dermatol.* 4:461, 1981.
5. Nemeth, A. Keloids and hypertrophic scars. *J Dermatol Surg Oncol.* 19:738–746, 1993.
6. Albom, MJ. Surgical gems: Dermo-subdermal sutures for long deep surgical wounds. *J Dermatol Surg Oncol.* 3:504–505, 1977.
7. Zitelli J, Moy R. Buried vertical mattress suture. *J Dermatol Surg Oncol.* 15:17–19, 1989.
8. Rook A, Wilkinson D, Ebling F (eds) et al. Textbook of Dermatology, 5th Ed., 1992, p. 3098.
9. Johnson JM, Ratner D, Nelson BR. Soft tissue reconstruction with skin grafting. *J Am Acad Dermatol.* 27:157, 1992.
10. Elson M. Effects of petroleum jelly on the healing of skin following cosmetic surgical procedures. *Cosmetic Dermatology.* 6:18–22, 1993.
11. Tromovitch TA, Stegman SJ, Glogau RG. Flaps and grafts in dermatologic surgery. *Mosby Year Book*; 1989:215–216.
12. Thompson SC, Jolley D, Marks R. Reduction of solar keratoses by regular sunscreen use. *N Engl J Med.* 329:1147–1151, 1993.
13. Australian Standard 2604. 1986 Sunscreen Products—Evaluation and Classification. Sydney, Standards Assoc. Australia, 1986.
14. Ryman W: Personal communication. NSW Skin and Cancer Foundation, (letter) Sydney, Australia, 1994.
15. Schreiber MM, Moon TE, Fox SH, et al. The risk of developing subsequent non-melanoma skin cancers. *J Am Acad Dermatol.* 23:1114–1118, 1990.
16. Green AC, O'Rourke MG. Cutaneous malignant melanoma in association with other skin cancers. *J Natl Cancer Inst.* 74:977–980, 1985.
17. Frank W, Rogers G. Melanoma update—second primary melanoma. *J Dermatol Surg Oncol.* 19:427–430, 1993.
18. Greene MH, Clarke WH, Tucker MA, Kraemer KH, Elder DE, Fraser ME. High risk of malignant melanoma in melanoma-prone families with dysplastic naevi. *Ann Int Med.* 102:458–465, 1985.
19. Lindelof B, Sigurgeirsson B, Wallberg P, et al. Occurrence of other malignancies in 1973: patients with basal cell carcinoma. *J Am Acad Dermatol.* 25:245–248, 1991.
20. Coldiron BM. Thinning of the ozone layer: Facts and consequences. *J Am Acad Dermatol.* 27:653–692, 1992.
21. Scotto J, Fears TR, Fraumeni JF. Incidence of nonmelanoma skin cancer in the United States. Bethesda, M.D. N.I.H. Publication No. 83-2433, 1984.

22. Marks R, Staples M, Giles GG. Trends in non-melanotic skin cancer treated in Australia: The second national survey. *Int J Cancer.* 53:585–590, 1993.

23. Kelly J, Marsden S, Sagebiel R. Frequency and duration of patient follow-up after treatment of a primary malignant melanoma. *J Am Acad Dermatol.* 13:756–760, 1985.

24. Scarborough D, Bisaccia A. The postoperative period: A rewarding yet critical time for both patient and dermatological surgeon. *Cosmetic Dermatology.* 5:8–10, 1993.

25. Bennett RG. Problems Associated with Cutaneous Surgery, in *Fundamentals of Cutaneous Surgery.* CV Mosby; pp 492–513, 1988.

26. Salasche SJ, Bernstein G. Surgical Anatomy of the Skin. Norwalk, Conn. Appleton and Lange; 1988:193.

27. Goldman M, Weiss R, Brody H, Coleman W, Fitzpatrick R. Treatment of facial telangiectasia with sclerotherapy, laser surgery, and/or electrodessication: A review. *J Dermatol Surg Oncol.* 19:899–906, 1993.

28. Barrett T, Greenway H, Massullo V, Carlson C. Treatment of basal cell carcinoma and squamous cell carcinoma with perineural invasion. *Adv Dermatol.* 8:277–305, 1993.

29. Summers BK, Siegle RJ. Facial cutaneous reconstructive surgery: General aesthetic principles. *J Am Acad Dermatol.* 29:669–681, 1993.

30. Kirscher CW, Shetlar MR, Shetlar CL. Alteration of hypertrophic scars induced by mechanical pressure. *Arch Dermatol.* 3:60–64, 1975.

31. Gold M. Topical silicone gel sheeting in the treatment of hypertrophic scars and keloids: A dermatologic experience. *J Dermatol Surg Oncol.* 19:912–916, 1993.

32. Burgess LPA, Morin GV, Rand M, Vossoughi J, Hollinger JA. Wound healing: Relationship of wound closing tension to scar width in rats. *Arch Otolaryngol Head Neck Surg.* 116:798–802, 1990.

33. Bennett RG. Problems associated with cutaneous surgery, in *Fundamentals of Cutaneous Surgery.* St Louis, MO: CV Mosby; 1988:506.

34. Tromovitch TA, Stegman SJ, Glogau RG. Flaps and grafts in dermatologic surgery. St Louis, MO: *Mosby Year Book*; 1989:216–217.

35. Katz BE, Oca MAGS. A controlled study of the effectiveness of spot dermabrasion ("scarabrasion") on the appearance of surgical scars. *J Am Acad Dermatol.* 24:462–466, 1991.

36. Salasche S, Bernstein G. Surgical anatomy of the skin. Norwalk: Appleton and Lange; 1988:170.

37. Salasche S, Bernstein G. Surgical anatomy of the skin. Norwalk: Appleton and Lange; 1988:37–44.

9

COMPLICATIONS

Christine M. Hayes, MD

Duane C. Whitaker, MD

INTRODUCTION

A complication from surgery can be defined as an unplanned event or events leading to a compromised cosmetic or functional outcome. This is also dependent on the patient's perception of the final result. Acceptability of outcome varies with the type of procedure performed. A patient may tolerate an obvious scar resulting from cancer surgery that would be an unacceptable result after a cosmetic procedure. Altered sensation or loss of motor function are unexpected after treatment of benign lesions but may be anticipated consequences in the treatment of malignancies.

Cutaneous surgery encompasses many procedures including biopsies, excisional surgery, Mohs' micrographic surgery, laser surgery, flaps, grafts, dermabrasion, and chemical peels. Surgical complications may be encountered including wound infection, hemorrhage, hematoma, dehiscence, necrosis, altered sensation, loss of motor function, and an unattractive scar. It is not always possible to identify an initiating event because hemorrhage and hematoma may lead to wound infection, necrosis of the wound edge, dehiscence, and finally an unattractive scar. The tetrad of hematoma, infection, dehiscence, and necrosis should alert the surgeon that when one is evident any of the remaining three may also be present or may follow.

PREVENTION

Inevitably, some complications will occur in a surgical practice. The goal of a preoperative evaluation is to maintain complications at the lowest rate possible.[1] A thorough preoperative evaluation can prevent many complications, and the risk and complexity of the planned procedure will dictate the extent of history and physical examination required. For biopsy or excisional procedures, awareness of pertinent past medical and surgical history, medications, and allergies is important. Large or multistaged procedures require a careful evaluation. Relevant medical history may include presence of artificial heart valves or joints, a detailed review of systems, history of any infectious bloodborne diseases, and social history. A social history is necessary to establish occupation, living situation, and high-risk behaviors, which may include smoking and intake of drugs or alcohol.

Host risk factors for surgical complications include diabetes, obesity, an immunocompromised state, and coincident infection at another site.[2] Smokers are at a higher risk for flap necrosis and overall poorer healing.[3] We have observed a higher complication rate in alcoholic patients. Further history regarding radiation, easy bleeding or bruising, slow healing, scarring, and difficulties with previous surgeries is significant.

Physical examination should include complete skin and oral mucosal examination and palpation of relevant lymph node sites. Quality of skin (sebaceous, acneiform, irradiated) and characteristics of personal hygiene should be noted. One should observe for lymphedema and obvious peripheral vascular disease, and examine previous surgical sites. Facial nerve function should be documented before any surgery on the face.

Various laboratory studies may be advisable in elderly and higher-risk patients, those with no history of previous surgery, and in large or complex cases. Complete blood count, including platelets, bleeding time, prothrombin time, and partial thromboplastin time, should be considered in the patient without previous surgical history. Serum chemistries, urinalysis, chest radiograph, or other imaging studies may be obtained if indicated by history or physical examination.

Discussion of possible complications and their management before surgery is a critical component of the informed consent process and will help prepare the patient for routine postoperative recovery. Details of transient edema, bruising, scar anesthesia, postoperative pain, temporary behavior modification, and patient responsibility for wound care should be addressed at the initial consultation.

WOUND INFECTION

Clean cutaneous surgery performed on healthy patients has a very low rate of wound infection (approximately 0.7%).[4] By far the most common infectious agents are bacteria, although infection due to viral, fungal, and parasitic agents may occasionally be seen. Most surgical wound infections are caused by *Staphylococcus aureus* organisms.[5,6] Moist body regions (groin, axillae, feet) are colonized by *Escherichia coli* and diphtheroids; cutaneous infections may be complicated by these organisms.[7]

An infected wound should be cultured and the empiric use of a penicillinase-resistant antibiotic is recommended. Therapy may then be altered when the organism and sensitivities are identified.

Wound infections appear clinically with erythema, warmth, and tenderness and may progress to fluctuation, purulence, and dusky wound edges. Figure 9-1 demonstrates erythema and induration at the surgical site on the forehead of an elderly patient. Vital signs should be taken and a complete blood count obtained to establish localization of the infection. If frank purulence is present, treatment consists of opening and culturing the wound, wound irrigation, and debridement of devitalized tissue. When purulence is evident, systemic antibiotics should be started. As infection in a diabetic can lead to diabetic ketoacidosis, a serum chemistry profile may be indicated with an obvious infection.

Clear-cut identification of a wound infection is often difficult. Many healing wounds are mildly erythematous and transiently indurated. If the culture shows no growth, does this negate the clinical suspicion of a wound infection? In epidemiologic studies, clinical signs of infection plus the clinician's decision to institute systemic antibiotics constitute a fairly reliable definition of infection.

Prophylactic antibiotics given in the preoperative period have been shown to decrease wound infection rates in clean-contaminated (violation of alimentary, respiratory, and genitourinary systems without spillage) and grossly contaminated (entered with spillage) surgical procedures. Skin surgery is considered a clean procedure, and the benefits of prophylaxis are not clear-cut. The patient at high risk for wound infection may be a candidate for prophylactic antibiosis. Administering antibiotics two hours before clean surgery has been shown to reduce the risk of wound infection.[8]

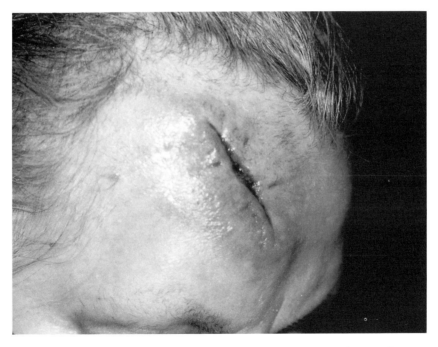

Figure 9.1. Forehead surgical defect with a wound infection in an elderly patient.

The most common viral agent seen postsurgically is herpes simplex type 1, which usually occurs in an abraded wound. Patients with large, denuded defects are at increased risk for postoperative herpes leading to severe scarring. It is therefore critical to determine a history of recurrent oral herpes simplex in patients considering dermabrasion, chemical peel, or facial laser surgery. Perioperative oral acyclovir may avoid this complication in patients at risk.

Candida albicans will occasionally cause a wound infection and is evidenced by white, pinpoint pustules studding the surface of a dusky, erythematous but nonpurulent wound. Figure 9-2 shows the upper lip of a woman with a cutaneous *Candida* infection at the surgical site.

Mycobacterium infection is rare, but contamination of tissue marking solution has been reported as an unusual source of wound infection in a plastic surgery practice.[9]

HEMORRHAGE/HEMATOMA

Hematoma formation may be due to coagulopathy (endogenous or acquired, most commonly through a drug[10]), inadequate coagulation of the vessels at the time of surgery, or patient noncompliance with postoperative instructions. Hypertension, anxiety, and ingestion of aspirin can complicate any of these etiologies. Prevention of hematoma is facilitated by elimination of dead space at the time of surgery. A pressure dressing is helpful in assisting coagulation. In areas where an effective pressure dressing is difficult

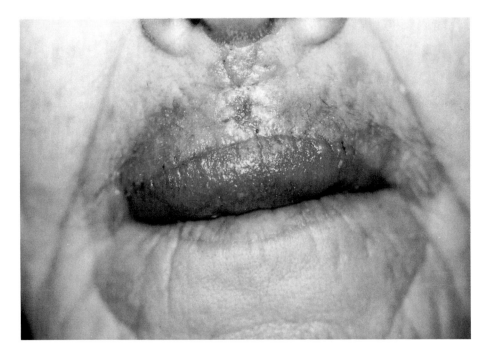

Figure 9.2. Upper lip with superficial *Candida albicans* infection after surgery.

to secure, ensuring adequate hemostasis is even more critical. Immobilization of the affected area may be necessary to prevent rebleeding in the early postoperative period.

Acute hematoma appears as a compressible mass in the area of the surgical site. It usually appears in the first 24 hours after surgery and nearly always within 72 hours. The patient may give a history of an expanding mass at the suture line. This is distinguished from an ecchymosis, which is blue-black, flat, and nonpalpable.

Evaluation of the patient presenting with a hematoma includes measurements of the heart rate, blood pressure, and hemoglobin/hematocrit if the volume of blood loss is indeterminant. If the blood loss appears significant, a peripheral access line should be started. Stabilization of vital signs, analgesia, and management of patient anxiety are essential first steps.

Hematoma evacuation is important because a hematoma is a nidus for infection, may apply pressure on vital structures, devitalize wound edges, or lead to flap or graft necrosis. Evacuation may be performed via a large-gauge needle if the hematoma is fluid or small and localized. If it is large or actively bleeding it may require anesthesia, reopening of the wound edges to thoroughly extract the hematoma, and cautery of bleeding vessels. Figure 9-3 shows a large hematoma that developed after surgery on the neck of an elderly man.

After hematoma extraction, a decision must be made to either pack the wound and allow second intention healing to ensue or to resuture the wound edges after adequate closure of the dead space. The classic teaching is that once the wound is reopened it should heal by second intention, but occasionally exceptions are made if there is no evi-

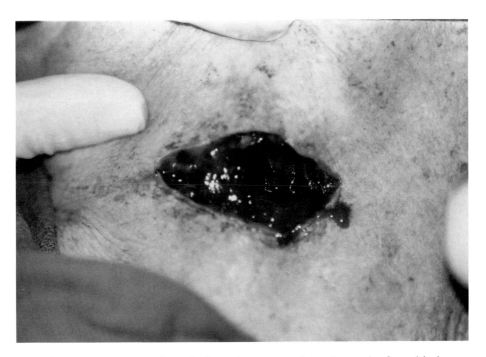

Figure 9.3. Evacuation of a large hematoma from the neck of an elderly man.

dence of contamination or necrosis. Immobilization of the area is critical to avoid dislodging microthrombi, which prevent recurrence of the hematoma. This may involve an effective pressure dressing and splinting to reduce movement. The neck is a difficult area to immobilize and is therefore an area of high risk for hematoma formation after surgery. Patients in whom immobilization is difficult or who have significant pain may require inpatient monitoring with analgesia and sedation. Medications and past medical and surgical history should be reviewed to seek contributing etiologies.

DEHISCENCE

Dehiscence or separation of the wound edges may occur as a primary or secondary complication. Causes include severe tension on the wound edges, wound infection, hematoma, and excessive movement of the affected body part. Tension on the wound edge can often be predicted at the time of closure by pallor or cyanosis. When the surgeon designs a layered or flap closure there should be little tension present. If pallor or duskiness is seen, the closure is too tight and the risk for dehiscence is heightened. Methods to decrease tension on the wound edge include alternative design of the flap, adequate undermining, and well-placed subcutaneous sutures. Figure 9-4 demonstrates dehiscence of wound edges on the forehead.

Excessive movement can be curtailed by an immobilizing dressing placed at the time of surgery. Limits on postoperative activity should always be reviewed with the patient before surgery.

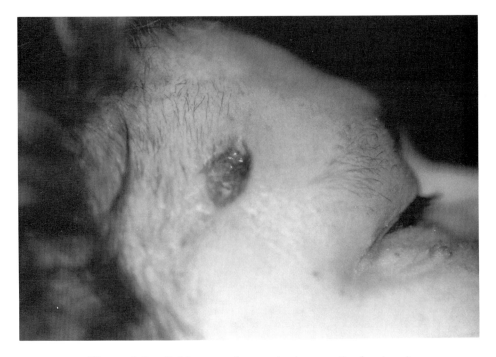

Figure 9.4.   Dehiscence of wound edges on the forehead.

When wound dehiscence does occur, constricting sutures are removed, and often the best management is through second-intention healing. In the short term the scar may be contracted and unsightly, but the long-term outcome can be satisfactory even without revision. Scar revision, if needed, should be approached only after the healing is complete (at least 6 to 12 months).

NECROSIS

In the healthy patient wound necrosis rarely occurs in isolation. Rather, it is usually a result of infection, hematoma, or constriction of blood supply to the tissue. Necrosis of the wound edges presents as dusky, violet, or gray skin edges, which may or may not be tender. Necrotic tissue requires debridement to avoid secondary infection. The latter is rarely seen in surgery on the head and neck unless sutures strangulate wound edges but is more common on the distal extremities. Figure 9-5 demonstrates necrotic tissue on the scalp.

Flap necrosis may occur at the tip or edge of a flap owing to tension on the wound edge. This is evident as a grayish area of the flap that does not regain a pink color with time. Assessment of partial necrosis requires experience, and pallid tissue should be preserved as it may be viable. Once demarcation of necrosis has occurred, judicious surgical débridement is required, with preservation of the viable portion of the flap. That area will then heal by second intention.

Necrosis of a full-thickness skin graft may occur if neovascularization does not

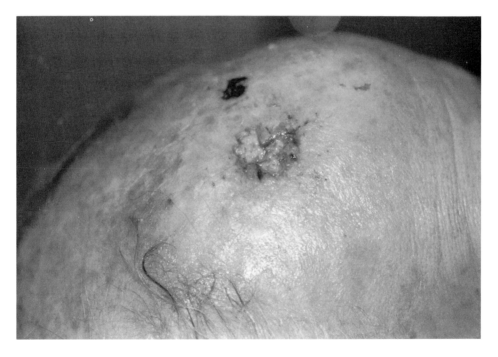

Figure 9.5.   Necrotic tissue on a scalp.

occur within 96 hours. Causes of graft necrosis include harvesting too large a graft for the recipient blood supply, inadequate defatting of the donor tissue, devascularized recipient bed, as in cartilage or bone lacking perichondrium or periosteum, hematoma formation under the graft, or inadequate apposition of the graft to the recipient bed. A graft that is black and dry is necrotic and should be debrided. However, a partially viable graft may appear dusky or violaceous and the portion that has taken is indeterminant. In these cases watching and waiting is recommended. Not uncommonly, the epidermis of a full-thickness skin graft will slough with the dermis intact. This is not a necrotic graft, and will remain viable and reepithelialize with time. As it may be difficult to assess graft viability in the first few weeks, extremely conservative debridement is recommended. Figure 9-6 shows a necrotic, nonviable, full-thickness skin graft.

If necrosis develops in the skin overlying cartilage or bone, the perichondrium or periosteum may become devitalized and expose the underlying tissue. In this event it is critical to keep the tissue moist, or death of the cartilage or bone may ensue. Necrotic cartilage appears dry and crumbles easily. Necrotic bone loses its sheen and appears desiccated. If this occurs, the necrotic tissue will require débridement.

ALTERED SENSATION FOLLOWING SURGERY

The patient will have decreased sensation directly on the scar line immediately after surgery. Sensation is usually regained unless a major branch of a sensory nerve is transected, and the patient should be counseled appropriately. In some cases, the slow regrowth of the nerves over 18 to 24 months results in at least partial sensory return.

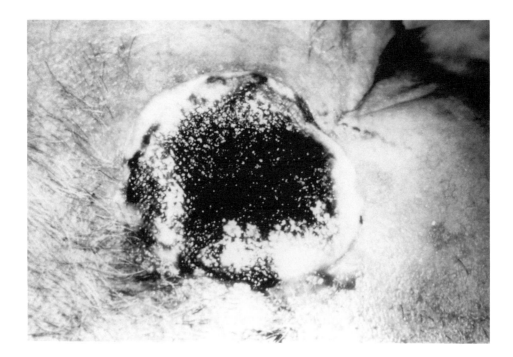

Figure 9.6.   Necrotic full-thickness skin graft.

Detailed discussion of facial anatomy is beyond the scope of this chapter, and reference to an excellent anatomy text should be sought.[11,12,13] However, the following points are of particular importance. When performing surgery in the vicinity of the great auricular nerve in the neck and the three divisions of the trigeminal nerve (ophthalmic, maxillary, and mandibular) in the face, there is greater risk of facial sensory nerve loss. Knowledge of cutaneous anatomy is critical; injury to these sensory nerves may result in profound and permanent cutaneous anesthesia.

The great auricular nerve supplies sensation to the earlobe, posterior auricle, inferior parotid area, and mastoid area. It exits the posterior border of the sternocleidomastoid and ascends to the earlobe. Injury to this nerve results in anesthesia superior to the point of transection.

The trigeminal nerve provides sensation to the face via its three divisions. A branch of the first division (ophthalmic), the supraorbital nerve, exits via the supraorbital foramen, located at the superior orbital rim in the midpupillary line. This nerve supplies sensation to the forehead and frontal scalp. The second division, maxillary, gives off the infraorbital nerve, which exits via the infraorbital foramen, located approximately 1 cm below the inferior orbital rim in the midpupillary line. This nerve supplies sensation to the cheek, lateral nose, and upper lip. A branch of the third division (maxillary), the mental nerve, exits via the mental foramen, located in the mandible in the midpupillary line. The mental nerve supplies sensation to the chin and lower lip. Injury to one of these nerves results in anesthesia of the area supplied.

LOSS OF MOTOR FUNCTION

The motor nerves most often at risk for injury in cutaneous surgery on the head and neck are the branches of cranial nerve VII (the facial nerve) and cranial nerve XI (spinal accessory).

The facial nerve provides motor function to the muscles of facial expression. Figure 9-7 shows the branches of the facial nerve. Injury to any of the branches will result in some loss of facial animation. In general, however, the temporal and marginal mandibular branches are most susceptible to injury during cutaneous surgical procedures. The temporal branch of cranial nerve VII exits the anterior margin of the parotid gland and is most superficial in the temple region. It provides motor function to the frontalis muscle and helps to raise the eyebrow and forehead. The marginal mandibular branch of cranial nerve VII courses along the inferior margin of the mandible and is superficial in the vicinity of the facial artery. It provides motor function to the muscles of facial expression and helps to smile, frown, and tightly close the lips. Figure 9-8 depicts facial hemiparesis following oncologic surgery.

The spinal accessory nerve exits from the deep posterior margin of the sternocleidomastoid muscle in an area called Erb's point. Erb's point can be found by drawing a horizontal line connecting the angle of the jaw and the mastoid process. From the midpoint of the line a vertical line is then dropped. Erb's point is the intersection of this vertical line with the posterior border of the sternocleidomastoid muscle. The spinal accessory nerve innervates the sternocleidomastoid muscle and then passes posteriorly to innervate the trapezius muscle. At its point of exit it is susceptible to injury and therefore extreme care must be taken when planning surgery in this region.

Facial Nerve Divisions

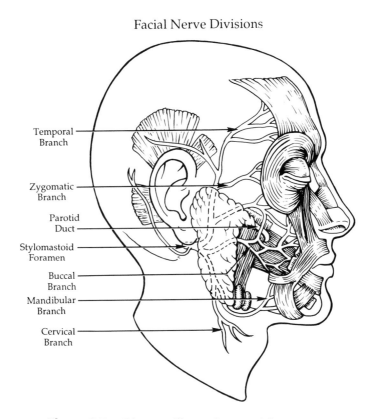

Temporal
Branch

Zygomatic
Branch

Parotid
Duct

Stylomastoid
Foramen

Buccal
Branch

Mandibular
Branch

Cervical
Branch

Figure 9.7.   Diagram illustrating cranial nerve VII.

ANESTHESIA

The major complications from anesthesia are related to allergic reactions and toxicity. There are very few patients who are truly allergic to local anesthetics though some may experience palpitations due to epinephrine. The ester class of anesthetics causes more allergic reactions[14]; however, lidocaine is of the amide type and is usually well tolerated.

Lidocaine in high serum concentrations causes toxic effects, mainly involving the central nervous system. Symptoms include dizziness, drowsiness, tinnitus, and perioral paresthesia.[14,15] At very high concentrations convulsions, coma, and cardiorespiratory arrest are seen. Therefore it is advisable to use the lowest dose necessary to induce anesthesia. Dangerously high serum levels leading to death have been reported in the use of lidocaine cream in large amounts on ulcerated skin.[15]

HYPERTROPHIC SCAR/KELOID

Spread of the scar following surgery is a common phenomenon.[16] In pediatric and adolescent patients it is often unavoidable. It should be predicted preoperatively and explained to the patient and parent. Careful surgical planning and technique may help

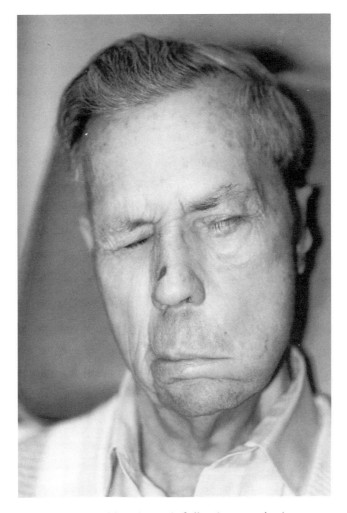

Figure 9.8. Facial hemiparesis following oncologic surgery.

to minimize scar spread. Sometimes scar maturation will yield an acceptable result, however scar revision in the future may ultimately be sought.

Some patients have a tendency to develop hypertrophic scars. The incidence of hypertrophy is higher in younger patients. A history of hypertrophic scarring increases the risk and should be discussed with the patient and his or her parents, who may choose to forego any elective surgery. Particular anatomic areas are at higher risk, including presternal and deltoid regions and the upper back. This is often a function of location and may not be due to the procedure or closure performed. Hypertrophy and keloid formation have a higher incidence in black and Asian patients.

Hypertrophic scars may flatten with time alone, though intralesional cortico-steroid injections may accelerate the process. Figure 9-9 shows corticosteroid injection into a hypertrophic scar. Keloids, by definition, are thickened scar tissues that extend

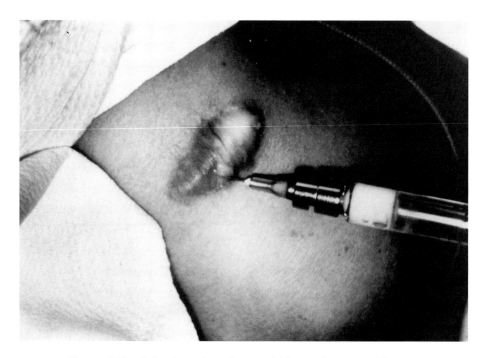

Figure 9.9. Injection of corticosteroid into a hypertrophic scar.

beyond the margins of the surgical scar. The importance of this distinction is the frequent lack of response to treatment in keloid scars. Keloids form in acne scars or surgical scars, most commonly in the presternal, deltoid, or scapular areas. Keloids can be very resistant to treatment, but conservative therapy such as compression dressings and intralesional corticosteroids can improve symptoms.[17] Although early reports suggested benefit from laser treatment of keloids, there is a high recurrence rate following either scalpel or laser surgical excision.[18] Such treatments are usually combined with intralesional corticosteroids. Recently, topical silicone gel has been used for prevention and treatment of hypertrophic scars.[19] Low-dose radiation has been reported[20] but is associated with long-term complications and is not recommended.

SCAR/DISFIGUREMENT

Any surgical procedure will result in a scar. However, scars can be minimized by camouflage, ie, the placement of the surgical scar in the natural lines of the face. This is more easily accomplished in the elderly, who have obvious relaxed skin tension lines (Langer's lines) or rhytides. Placement of a scar parallel to the relaxed skin tension lines will disguise it; conversely, a scar that is perpendicular to the relaxed skin tension lines will be more obvious.

A second important concept is recognition of facial cosmetic units such as the cheek, nose, lips, and chin.[12] If a scar can be kept within one cosmetic unit it is less noticeable than if it crosses units. Also, placing a scar in a junction between facial units, such as the melolabial fold, will make it less conspicuous.

An oncologic surgical procedure may lead to an unpredictable and larger defect than one involving a benign lesion. If surgery leads to the alteration or loss of a normal structure on the face, such as an eyebrow or nose, deformity will result. In such instances reconstructive procedures or prosthetic devices may in part, but not entirely, replace function and cosmesis. Figure 9-10 demonstrates a disfiguring scar after oncologic surgery and maxillectomy. Deformity should be anticipated, the patient appropriately counseled, and ancillary services consulted. Patients with extensive facial tumors may require prosthetic consultation before surgery. Figure 9-11 shows the same patient wearing a prosthetic device.

Some patients will require extensive counseling and psychological support for facial surgery. This does not always correlate with the severity of the surgery but rather

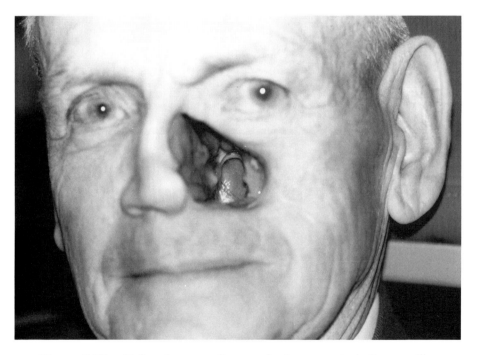

Figure 9.10.   Disfiguring scar after oncologic surgery including maxillectomy. Note: Camera focus is on base of defect.

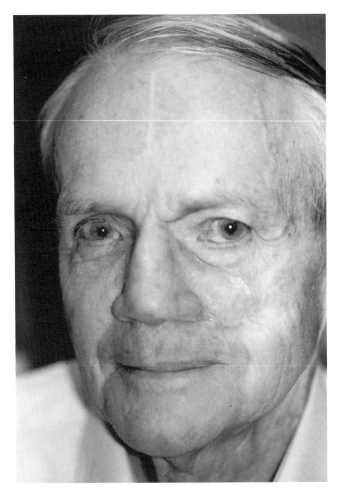

Figure 9.11.   Same patient wearing prosthetic device.

with patient concern and psychological makeup. The cosmetic appearance of the scar can vary depending on its location on the body and the patient's skin characteristics. Scar contraction that inhibits facial movement should be revised when possible. Less severe scarring is sometimes self-correcting by maturation of the scar tissue. Scar revision may involve intralesional corticosteroid injections, dermabrasion (scarabrasion), excision of the scar and closure with a less obvious surgical wound, or a combination of these techniques.

CONTACT DERMATITIS

This is not a rare complication after surgery and may be mistaken for a wound infection by the nondermatologist. The most common offenders are adhesives and topical antibiotics. Adhesives often cause erythema or vesiculation in a telltale rectangular pattern, as seen in Figure 9-12. It is more difficult to diagnose a dermatitis due to antibiotic ointment, as it appears with subtle erythema, induration, or delayed healing. The erythema may simulate an early wound infection and not respond to antibiotics. Polymyxin B sulfate/bacitracin zinc ointment with neomycin is a common offender; polymyxin B sulfate/bacitracin zinc ointment is less common but not rare. Treatment consists of discontinuing the offending agent and beginning an alternative ointment, such as mupiricin or bacteriostatic emollient.

CHONDRITIS

Chondritis or perichondritis may occur when surgery is performed on the ear or nose. Cartilage exposure or disruption can result in erythema, edema, and pain at the site of surgery. Figure 9-13 demonstrates chondritis of the auricle. Clinically, it may appear to be of combined etiology—chondritis and infection. If symptomatic, this is best treated by culture, antibiotics, local heat and the administration of nonsteroidal, anti-inflammatory medications for pain. If the wound shows evidence of necrotic or friable cartilage this should be debrided.[21] An important consideration must be to exclude malignant otitis externa, a severe infection caused by *Pseudomonas aeruginosa* that appears as a chronically draining otitis of the external ear and may involve the entire auricle with extension into bone.

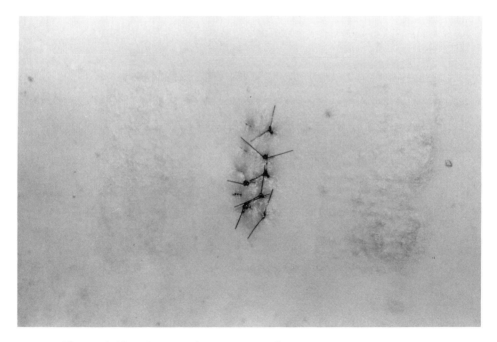

Figure 9.12.   Contact dermatitis to adhesive applied to suture line.

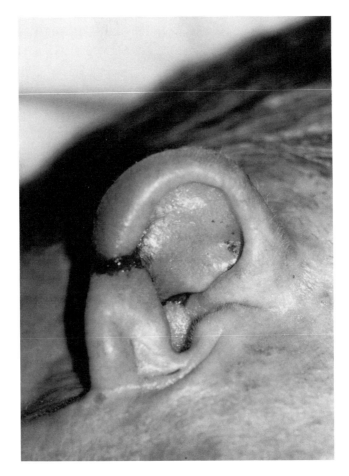

Figure 9.13.   Chondritis following wedge excision on the auricle.

MINOR COMPLICATIONS

Hypertrophic granulation tissue may develop along the margins of a wound healing by second intention. This is usually transient and may resolve with desiccation of the wound bed. If it does not, cauterization with silver nitrate sticks or excision may be necessary.

Rarely after surgery pyogenic granulomas can develop in the surgical site. Treatment consists of adequate removal of all lesions. Patients on systemic retinoid therapy may be predisposed to the development of pyogenic granuloma–like lesions.[22]

Buried sutures placed in the subcutaneous or dermal tissue may not be absorbed and instead may extrude through the wound during the healing process (spitting suture). This complication is usually minor and in the absence of infection almost never compromises the final outcome. It usually occurs between weeks two and eight after surgery and is more common with larger-diameter suture buried superficially. One can minimize the problem by burying the knots of the subcutaneous suture deeply and limiting the amount of suture material buried.

Hyperpigmentation is a very common but transient side effect of surgery. Sunscreens and hydroquinone products are useful in assisting the natural fading of hyperpigmentation.

Hypopigmentation, particularly following cryosurgery, tends to be longer lasting and can be permanent if there is significant injury to melanocytes. Pigmentary irregularities may be more noticeable in dark-skinned patients and therefore cause greater cosmetic concern.

Milia are white, pinpoint epidermal inclusion cysts. They are commonly seen in the treated areas after dermabrasion but can be seen along suture incision lines. They are easily removed by lancing the epidermis with a #11 blade and expressing the cyst contents with a comedo extractor.

Postoperative seroma is a localized collection of serum that appears as a compressible, nontender, nonerythematous swelling and tends to occur later in the course of wound healing. The most common setting is a healed wound with an area of dead space or under a mature skin graft. Treatment consists of evacuation with a large-gauge needle followed with a compression dressing, although small seromas may resolve with time and pressure alone.

PATIENT EXPECTATIONS

Preoperative consultation and evaluation is necessary before a surgical procedure beyond minor biopsy. The approach varies with procedures of medical necessity versus elective surgery. Every patient should understand the procedure he or she is about to undergo, the risks, and the likely outcome. The physician should assess patient expectations and determine if they are realistic. Planned excision of a benign lesion allows the patient to weigh the benefits and outcome with the risks of the procedure. Often the unhappy patient had unrealistic expectations initially but was not dissuaded of them.

Before oncologic surgery, patients may be anxious and, though they understand the necessity of surgery, not appreciative of the magnitude of potential surgical and reconstructive outcome. Education of spouse and family can help the oncology patient cope with his or her responsibilities in the recovery process. Cosmetic procedures require a somewhat different approach, because expectations are often high. Initial consultation before elective cosmetic procedures should allow sufficient time for explanation and questions.

When evaluating a patient who has an acceptable scar but is unhappy with the result, it is important to listen to the patient's concerns, remain empathetic, and objectively assess the surgical outcome without becoming defensive. Allow the patient hope that something can be done to improve the scar if he or she remains displeased. In oncologic surgery, remind the patient of the beneficial aspects, that is, tumor eradication and possible worse outcome had treatment been delayed. It is important that the dissatisfied patient not feel abandoned; therefore continuity of care is critical. Finally, consider that there may be more than meets the eye and the true problem may actually be unrelated to the surgery. The patient may focus on a surgical scar as the source of present frustrations in life. The spouse's perception may also be useful.

SUMMARY

There are many complications that may develop when performing surgical procedures. With adequate preoperative preparation and careful technique they will be kept to a minimum. Knowledge beforehand of the possible difficulties will enable the surgeon to recognize them when encountered and will lead to appropriate management.

REFERENCES

1. Leshin B, McCalmont TH. Preoperative evaluation of the surgical patient. *Dermatol Clin.* 8:787–794, 1990.
2. Wenzel RP. Preoperative antibiotic prophylaxis. *N Engl J Med.* 326:337–338, 1992.
3. Goldminz D, Bennett RG. Cigarette smoking and flap and full thickness graft necrosis. *Arch Dermatol.* 127:1012–1015, 1991.
4. Whitaker DC, Grande DJ, Johnson SS. Wound infection rate in dermatologic surgery. *J Dermatol Surg Oncol.* 14:525–528, 1988.
5. Jarvis WR, Martone WJ. Predominant pathogens in hospital infections. *J Antimicrob Chemo.* 29(Suppl A):19–24, 1992.
6. Twum-Danso K, Grant C, Al-Suleiman SA, et al. Microbiology of postoperative wound infection: A prospective study of 1770 wounds. *J Hosp Infect.* 21:29–37, 1991.
7. Leyden JJ, McGinley KJ, Nordstrom KM, et al. Skin microflora. *J Invest Dermatol.* 88:65s–72s, 1987.
8. Classen DC, Evans RS, Pestotnik SL, et al. The timing of prophylactic administration of antibiotics and the risk of surgical-wound infection. *N Engl J Med.* 326:281–286, 1992.
9. Safranek TJ, Jarvis WR, Carson LA, et al. Mycobacterium Chelonae wound infections after plastic surgery employing contaminated gentian violet skin-marking solution. *N Engl J Med.* 317:197–201, 1987.
10. Bork K. *Cutaneous Side Effects of Drugs.* Philadelphia, PA: WB Saunders; 1988:194.
11. McMinn RMH, Hutchings RT, Logan BM. *Color Atlas of Head and Neck Anatomy.* Chicago, IL: YearBook Medical Publishers, Inc.; 1981:94–99, 112–113, 118–119.
12. Salasche SJ, Bernstein G, Senkarik M. *Surgical Anatomy of the Skin.* Norwalk, CT: Appleton and Lange; 1988:99–125.
13. Netter FH. *Atlas of Human Anatomy.* Summit, NJ: Ciba-Geigy Corporation; 1989:18–21, 26–27.
14. Auletta MJ, Grekin RC. *Local Anesthesia for Dermatologic Surgery.* New York, NY: Churchill Livingstone; 1991:14–16.
15. Lie RL, Vermeer BJ, Edelbroek PM. Severe lidocaine intoxication by cutaneous absorption. *J Am Acad Dermatol.* 23:1026–1028, 1990.
16. Bennett RG. *Fundamentals of Cutaneous Surgery.* St Louis, MO: CV Mosby; 1988:502.
17. Brown LA, Pierce HE. Keloids: Scarrevision. *J Dermatol Surg Oncol.* 12:51–56, 1986.
18. Apfelberg DB, Maser MR, White DN, et al. Failure of carbon dioxide laser excision of keloids. *Lasers Surg Med.* 9:382–388, 1989.
19. Ahn ST, Monafo WW, Mustoe TA. Topical silicone gel for the prevention and treatment of hypertrophic scar. *Arch Surg.* 126:499–504, 1991.

20. Borok TL, Bray M, Sinclair I, et al. Role of ionizing irradiation for 393 keloids. *Int J Radiol Oncol Biol Phys.* 15:865–870, 1988.
21. Larson PO, Ragi G, Mohs FE, et al. Excision of exposed cartilage for management of Mohs surgery defects of the ear. *J Dermatol Surg Oncol.* 17:749–752, 1991.
22. Exner JH, Dahod S, Pochi PE. Pyogenic granuloma-like acne lesions during isotretinoin therapy. *Arch Dermatol.* 119:808–811, 1983.

10

PRESURGICAL AND POSTSURGICAL NURSING

Judith A. Plis, BS, MBA

Nancy L. Vargo, RN

During the course of preparing a patient for surgery, there are several steps that should be followed that concern the nurse-to-patient information interchange. The nurse will discuss with the patient what can be expected both before and after surgery and obtain all the medication history and social history of the patient.

PREOPERATIVE CONSULTATION

Ideally, a preoperative consultation is scheduled for all patients before any dermatologic surgical procedure. During this appointment, the physician has an opportunity to discuss with the patient and his or her family the diagnosis and the treatment recommendation.

In a collaborative practice, the nurse also plays several key roles during this consultation period. There may be special arrangements before the patient's visit including advice about scheduling, requesting (or arranging for) necessary laboratory and pathology data, or assessing the need for interpreters for those patients unable to understand English.

Once the patient concludes the consultation, the nurse will meet with the patient and family to discuss any additional questions and reiterate information already provided by the physician. This interview with the patients will provide the nurse an opportunity to assess the patient's understanding of the disease and his or her perception of the treatment recommendation. Additionally, the nurse will assess patient expectation and understanding of the surgery being planned. Any discrepancies regarding patient expectations should be brought to the attention of the physician.

Patients with cutaneous malignancies will be anxious relating to their diagnosis of cancer, and they may only hear half of what is being said to them during that initial visit. They may be fearful of many things, including pain, disfigurement, and the possibility that a particular lesion may recur. Some patients may not ask any questions because they feel they will be better off not knowing what will take place during a particular procedure and therefore nothing bad will happen to them. Other patients may be very vocal about their feelings and relate their fears to the nurse, who should in turn inform the physician.

Cosmetic surgery patients have similar needs and will do much better on their surgical date if they, too, have clear expectations[1]. Nurses can provide valuable information by helping to produce patient education handouts, photographs, or videos to supplement the consultation. The nurses are the ones who will be tending to the patient the majority of the time that the patient is in the physician's office and the surgical arena.

During that consultation the nurse would also provide information about the following considerations:

a. What the patient can expect on the day of surgery
b. What preoperative preparations the patient will need to undertake
c. The length of time the procedure will take and how long the patient will be in the office on the day of surgery
d. The degree of sedation, if any, and if the patients have someone with them to drive them to and from the office
e. What type of dressing will be used
f. How long the healing time will be and when they can expect to have a normal appearance at the surgical site
g. When they can wear makeup
h. A general review of the procedure the physician has outlined and assisting the patient in its understanding.
i. How long will the patient need to be out of work and other activity restrictions they may expect

Depending on the surgical recommendation, some patients may require the services of other members of the health care team such as a facial plastic reconstruction physician, plastic surgeon, occuloplastic surgeon, or other physicians. Often, procedures that require a team approach may be performed in the operating suite under general anesthesia. These patients may anticipate admission to the hospital or an outpatient surgical center for preoperative work more extensive than that required for an office surgical procedure.

It is the nurse that patients will look to for reassurance and guidance during an unsettling and trying time. Patients may not fully understand what they may look like or how they may feel after a procedure has been performed. It is up to the nursing staff to make sure that patients feel comfortable and reassure them that everything necessary will be done to ensure that they receive the best care possible. The nursing staff will also be responsible for the following preoperative and postoperative assessments.

PREOPERATIVE ASSESSMENT

What is the patient's expectation and understanding of the procedure that he or she is about to undergo? Does the patient understand the procedure that is about to be performed? The nurses will make sure that the physician has adequately explained the procedure to the patient and if the patient still has any doubts as to the procedure being performed, then the nurse should have the physician return to see the patient and review the procedure again.

How anxious is the patient? The nurse tending to patients will assess how anxious and apprehensive he or she is. The nurse will also provide information and an explanation again to the patient, as to what they may expect. The nurse explains to the patients what will be taking place during a particular procedure. The equipment in the room should also be explained to help relieve any fears and anxiety that the patient may have while surveying the room. If the nurse feels that the patient may benefit from some preoperative sedation, then the nurse needs to alert the physician, who may order a sedative. Some patients, such as the elderly or those with liver, thyroid, central nervous system, pulmonary disease, anemia, are sensitive to even low doses of sedatives. Other patients, such as those patients who regularly use sedatives or alcoholic beverages or are extremely anxious, may require higher doses.

HEALTH ASSESSMENT

The health assessment may be performed by the physician or nurse, and often both collaborate on this vital aspect of the assessment. A knowledgeable assessment will provide an opportunity for timely intervention in the health problems of patients who may be at risk during surgery or who require special preoperative medications or precautions. It is often the nurse who will document this assessment and may rely on an assessment tool. (Figure 10-1).

MEDICATION HISTORY

The nurse will ask the patient what medications he or she takes on a regular basis. This will provide insight into any health problems the patient may be experiencing. The nurse needs to record all of the medication allergies that the patient has and to alert the physician, especially if the patient has had a sensitivity to any local anesthesia in the past (Figure 10-2).

All current medications that the patient is using need to be listed. It is important to know if the patient is taking anticoagulants, as this may lead to prolonged intraoperative or postoperative bleeding which could lead to the formation of a hematoma and delayed wound healing. The nurse should have the patient check with his or her pri-

SCRIPPS CLINIC
AND RESEARCH FOUNDATION

Nursing Notes
MINOR PROCEDURE

Patient Name: _____

Record #: _____

Date _____ Inpatient _____ Outpatient _____ Doctor _____

Pre-procedure vitals _____ Dentures _____

Consent signed _____ (G.I. consent to be signed in that department)

Drug allergies _____

CURRENT MEDS	Yes or No	Last Taken
Coumadin		
Insulin		
Antibiotics		
Digoxin		
Steroids		
Other		

DISEASES	Yes or No
Diabetes	
Heart	
Asthma	
Bleeding tendencies	
Emboli	
Hepatitis	
Glaucoma	
Other	

Last ate _____

Pre-procedure meds _____

Signature of the nurse completing above _____

PROCEDURE _____

Started _____ Ended _____

Medications: route/site/time/Doctor/or signature.

_____
_____
_____
_____

Specimen obtained _____

Specimen disposition _____

Post Vital signs _____

REMARKS _____

_____
_____
_____
_____
_____
_____

Signature _____

Figure 10.1.   Minor procedure form used in dermatologic surgery.

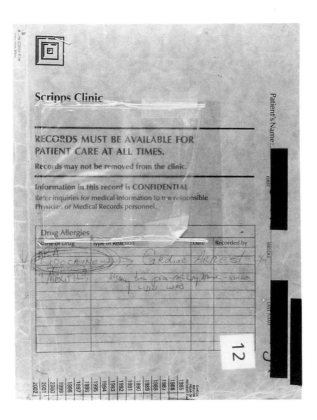

Figure 10.2.   Patient chart with patient allergy clearly labeled as below:

Name of Drug   **Type of Reaction**

Lidocaine   Cardiac arrest

The nurse should clearly investigate this chart before any
dermatologic surgical procedure.

mary physician before discontinuing any prescribed anticoagulant medications including aspirin, persantine, or coumadin.[2,3,4,5] If acceptable with the patient's physician,
have the patient discontinue aspirin 10 to 14 days before and one day after surgery and
discontinue warfarin (coumadin) four days before and one day after surgery. Also have
the patient discontinues any nonsteroidal, anti-inflammatory medications and switches
to acetaminophen if possible.

Certain medications may react with local anesthesia; it is important to know the
interactions of these medications and their effect on the patient. Propranolol (Inderal)
may cause malignant hypertension and bradycardia when used in conjunction with

lidocaine mixed with epinephrine.[6] In certain cases the physician may dilute the epinephrine. The patient's vital signs should be monitored during the procedure.

Diuretics (especially if taken with digitalis) can potentiate hypokalemia if the patient is given epinephrine in lidocaine.[6]

Immunosuppressive agents, such as prednisone, and antineoplastic drugs may delay wound healing.[2]

Neuroleptic agents such as phenothiazine (compazine, phenergan, stelazine, thorazine) and tricyclic antidepressants (elavil, triavil, amitril) may affect the patient's blood pressure and pulse.[6] MAO inhibitors (nardil, eutonyl, patnate) may result in a hypertensive crisis when used with epinephrine.[3,7]

MEDICAL HISTORY

Cardiac History

When a patient has a history of cerebral vascular accident or myocardial infarct, one needs to be aware that if epinephrine is used it will stimulate the cardiovascular system.[3] High blood levels of lidocaine may cause hypotension, cardiac depression manifested as prolonged conduction time, A-V block, and bradycardia.

Angina

Patients with angina may experience pain during the administration of local anesthetic or surgery. The physician may dilute the epinephrine with lidocaine. Sublingual nitroglycerin should be kept on the unit. The patient should also be instructed to bring his or her own nitroglycerin with them.

Arrhythmias

Patients that have arrhythmias may be at risk for dysrhythmia when lidocaine with epinephrine is used.

Pacemaker

When a patient has a pacemaker installed, short bursts of low current (less than five seconds) should be used when using an electrical cautery unit. A bipolar unit may be used with patients with a pacemaker[2,3] (see Chapter 1).

It is important that certain patients with the preceding conditions are placed on a cardiac monitor and that they are closely observed.

Patients with a history of valve disease,[3] such as mitral valve, prosthetic valves, congenital heart defect, coarctation of aorta, tetralogy of Fallot, or Marfan syndrome; infective endocarditis; mitral valve or tricuspid valve prolapse; pulmonary valve disease; asymmetric septal hypertrophy; or rheumatic heart disease may require antibiotic prophylaxis (see Chapter 1) for cutaneous surgical procedures.

Patients with hypertension may have an exaggerated response to epinephrine with lidocaine that may cause their blood pressure to become dangerously elevated.

Patients with a history of arthritis need to be asked when they last used non-steroidal anti-inflammatories and when they last used aspirin. Were they able to discontinue these medications before surgery as suggested?

Patients with prosthetic joints such as hip replacement (see Chapter 1) may need prophylactic antibiotics. The patients usually know that they have to take antibiotics before any dental or other surgical procedures, but the physician needs to ask to be sure that they indeed did take their medication.

Patients with diabetes may have impaired healing and antibiotics may be a postoperative consideration.

In patients with a history of peripheral vascular disease, the use of epinephrine in lidocaine may result in ischemic injury or necrosis.

Hyperthyroid patients may receive a cardiac stimulant effect from the epinephrine in lidocaine.

Patients with a history of a bleeding disorder may require preoperative labs (c.b.c., platelet count, peripheral smears, pro-time) and a good history.

In patients with a history of liver/kidney disease there could be lidocaine accumulation, and toxicity may occur due to impaired metabolism and the excretion of lidocaine. Impaired wound healing may also occur with liver disease.[2]

Patients with a history of a seizure disorder may need seizure precautions, and the lidocaine may need to be diluted.

Patients with narrow-angle glaucoma may not be at risk if the disease is well controlled; however, it may be advisable to dilute the epinephrine in lidocaine solution in certain cases.

Patients who are pregnant should be referred to the OB physician to be sure that they will be able to have the procedure. If the patients get clearance then it is best to perform the procedure toward the end of the pregnancy whenever possible. In some cases one may wait until after the delivery to perform the procedure.

Patients with a history of wound-healing problems, infection, keloid formation, or hypertrophic scarring may need special care. Immunosuppressed patients may have impaired wound healing and are at risk for infection and other complications.[2] Certain medications, such as corticosteroid or antineoplastic agents, may interfere with wound healing and increase the risk for infection.

Nursing Intervention

Alert the physician when the patients have any of the above conditions; preoperative and postoperative antibiotics may be prescribed. If the patient is currently having any problems with infection, the surgery may have to be rescheduled.

SOCIAL HISTORY

A social history should be obtained regarding the patient's living environment, support of family and friends, and communication or transportation difficulties. A history of alcohol or sedative use should also be noted. In addition, patients who smoke may experience impaired healing due to the vasoconstrictive effects of the nicotine.

INFORMED CONSENT

The physician is responsible for providing the information on the procedure to the patient, and the nurse may obtain the patient's signature and witness the document (Figure 10-3). The informed consent should be written with readability in mind, and in most cases, it should be written at a seventh- or eighth-grade level so that all patients can understand it. If the patient is a minor, then the signature of the parent or guardian will be required. If the patient is an emancipated minor then court documents need to be provided.

If the patient is unable to sign owing to severe arthritis or paraplegia then he or she may be able to mark the consent with an X. The witness may write "patient unable to sign owing to arthritis, and has read the above document and agrees verbally to undergo the procedure." This signature should also be witnessed. If the patient is mentally impaired then a guardian's signature is needed. If the patient arrives from an institution then they should arrive with a signed, dated consent from his or her legal guardian.

VITAL SIGNS

The nurses will assess the patient's vital signs at the beginning of any surgical procedure. If the patient is to undergo a more extensive surgical procedure then he or she may need to have full vital signs (such as blood pressure and pulse) read. If the patient has an elevated pressure or pulse, then he or she needs to have the pressure retaken in another position. If the pressure was taken while the patient was sitting, then the reading should be taken again while the patient is in a prone position, and further assessment regarding the patient's medical condition needs to be completed. The patient may just be nervous because of the impending surgery or have a medical condition that is elevating his or her blood pressure. Surgery may have to be delayed until the cause is found. In some cases a tranquilizer is all that is necessary to bring the patient's pressure down. In other cases the patient needs to see his or her primary physician and have blood pressure regulated before proceeding with the surgery. It is a good idea to put such a patient on a blood pressure monitor during the procedure so that his or her pressure can be monitored at regular intervals. If the patient has a history of heart problems and has a pacemaker then he or she should be put on a heart monitor as well.

It may be necessary to obtain the patient's temperature if he or she comes in with a cold or complain of any flulike symptoms. If the temperature is elevated then the physician does an assessment as to whether to proceed with the operation.

PREOPERATIVE SEDATION

The physician and the nurse will assess the patient's anxiety level and the possible need for preoperative sedatives. Valium (diazepam) is the agent we prefer to be administered postoperatively, SL (sublingually), or by I.V.[1] Valium produces a mild to moderate calming effect. Intravenous administration provides more intense levels of sedation, but caution needs to be exercised with the elderly or debilitated patient. Intravenous administration is more likely to produce respiratory depression.[3] Intravenous valium should

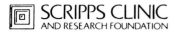 SCRIPPS CLINIC
AND RESEARCH FOUNDATION

**AUTHORIZATION FOR AND CONSENT TO SURGERY, ANESTHESIA
OR SPECIAL DIAGNOSTIC OR THERAPEUTIC PROCEDURES**

TO: _____

Your admitting physician is _____, M.D.

Your surgeon is _____, M.D.

1.   The clinic maintains personnel and facilities to assist your physicians and surgeons in their performance of various surgical operations and other special diagnostic and therapeutic procedures. These surgical operations and special diagnostic and therapeutic procedures all may involve calculated risks of complications, injury or even death, from both known and unknown causes and no warranty or guarantee has been made as to result or cure. Except in cases of emergency or exceptional circumstances, these operations and procedures are therefore not performed upon patients unless and until the patient has had an opportunity to discuss them with his physician. Each patient has the right to consent to or refuse any proposed operation or special procedure based upon the description or explanation received.

2.   Your physicians and surgeons have determined that the operations or special procedures listed below may be beneficial in the diagnosis or treatment of your condition. Upon your authorization and consent, such operations or special procedures will be performed for you by your physicians or surgeons and/or by other physicians and surgeons selected by them. The persons in attendance for the purpose of administering anesthesia may not be agents, servants or employees of the clinic or your physicans or surgeons, but may be independent contractors performing specialized services on your behalf and, as such, would be your agents, servants or employees. Any removed tissue, member or fluid will be disposed of at the discretion of the pathologist, except _____

_____
Any removed tissue or fluid may be used for scientific research or other investigational purpose but only if that research has received the approval of the Human Research Committee of the Scripps Clinic and Research Foundation. Such use will not alter the surgical or anesthetic procedure normally followed.

3.   Your signature below the operations or special procedures listed below constitutes your acknowledgment that you have read and agreed to the foregoing, that the operations or special procedures have been adequately explained to you by your attending physicians or surgeons and that you have all the information that you desire, and that you authorize and consent to the performance of the operations or special procedures. Your signature also indicates that you understand risks of having or not having the operation or procedure listed, the possible benefits of this procedure, that complications are possible, and the alternative forms of treatment.

Operation or procedure: _____

_____

_____

_____

Signed _____   Date _____

Witness _____   Time _____ am/pm

Patient is a minor, or unable to sign because _____

I hereby consent to the above operation or procedure for my _____

Signed _____   Date _____

Relationship _____   Time _____ am/pm

Witness _____

Physician's Risks and Alternatives Statement

_____

_____

_____

_____

131R286   Signed _____ M.D.   Date _____

Figure 10.3.   Sample of informed consent.

be administered slowly to reduce the possibility of pain, phlebitis, or venous thrombo-sis at the injection site.

Versed (midazalam) administered through deep I.M. or I.V. is twice as potent as Valium, producing better sedation and amnesia. Versed has a fast onset of action, a shorter half-life than Valium, and less likelihood of venous complications.[5] The nurse should ensure that the patient not drive until the day after procedure. There is an increased risk of apnea when the drug is given along with a narcotic premedication. The physician may order supplemental oxygen, and midazalam should be used with caution in the elderly and patients with chronic obstructive pulmonary, hepatic, or renal dis-ease. The FDA has warned of potential respiratory arrest with this drug; respiratory depression is not reversed by Naloxone (an opioid antagonist). Monitoring of the blood pressure is required, and the patient needs to be watched for hypotension.

Chloral hydrate may be a more effective sedative for the elderly and children. It is relatively safe, but may produce nausea and vomiting if given on an empty stomach.[3,4]

Preoperative opioid analgesics are often prescribed for complex procedures. Narcotics should be avoided for patients with respiratory disease. These drugs may pro-duce nausea, vomiting, hypotension, and respiratory depression lasting several hours. Narcan (Naloxone) and resuscitation equipment must be available on the unit.[8]

Morphine given I.M., subcutaneous (SQ) produces sedation, analgesia, and a feel-ing of euphoria. The nurse should be aware that the patient may experience nausea and respiratory depression.

Demerol (meperidine) administered I.M. or SQ produces analgesia and sedation with less euphoria than morphine. Side effects include dryness of the mouth, flushed face, diaphoresis, and emesis. This drug is often used in combination with Vistaril. Demerol may produce respiratory depression lasting up to four hours.

Sublimaze (fentanyl) given I.M. or I.V. is a potent synthetic narcotic analgesic with less likelihood of producing nausea or vomiting. It has a short duration of action but may cause respiratory depression, with excessive dosages producing apnea. There may be central-nervous-system depression in patients receiving tranquilizers and other nar-cotics or barbiturates.[9]

INTRAOPERATIVE ASSESSMENT

Patient comfort and safety during the procedure is as important as the preoperative and postoperative assessment performed by the nursing personnel.

Positioning of the patient is important for his or her comfort and well-being. If the patient is comfortable then the physician and staff will have an easier time performing the procedure.

In most cases you will have the patient lie down before injection of local anesthe-sia. Be sure there is a pillow that is in a comfortable position underneath the patient's head; there should also be one under the patient's knees to support his or her back.

Most procedures in cutaneous surgery are performed with only a local anesthetic. The patient is apprehensive and aware of your actions but may not understand fully. Be sure that you tell the patient when you are putting on surgical drapes so that he or she will know exactly what you are doing. The patient may be given an eye test (visual acuity) before any surgery around the eye. If you need to use an eye shield be sure to explain to the patient what it is and why you are using it. You also need to be sure that the patient has not had cataract surgery, a lens implant, or any eye disease before you use an eye shield. Touch is very important to the patient, especially if the eyes are covered. A hand touching an arm or a gentle pat will help reassure the patient. Having music in the room can help the patient to relax and take his or her mind off of what is happening. If a patient has been premedicated, then that patient needs to have a safety strap in place so that he or she doesn't inadvertently roll off the surgery table. If the patient needs to be left alone in the room for any reason be sure that the patient's eyes are uncovered, the safety strap is in place, and the table is in the lowest position possible. Always tell the patient where you are going and that you or one of the other nursing staff will be checking on him or her.

During the procedure the nurse will assess the patient's tolerance. Does the patient seem anxious or nervous? The nurse can visually assess the patient as he or she lies on the table and can generally tell if the patient needs to have further local anesthetic. The nurse will also monitor the vital signs and medications or I.V. fluids given.

Monitoring may involve observing the patient for signs of stress or staying with the patient if he or she is receiving I.V. medications.

COMPLICATIONS

Complications can and do arise during any procedure. When this happens physicians must not say "oops" or unnecessarily talk out loud, as the patients are awake and can hear everything. Physicians need to remain calm and attend to the situation at hand.

The patient experiences a drop in blood pressure due to involuntary internal responses and will be pale, diaphoretic and may complain of feeling nauseated or faint. In which case the patient should be immediately put into an Trendelenburg's position.[2] Then the nurse should assess the vital signs, and place a cool washcloth on the patient's forehead and neck. Ammonia capsules and oxygen should also be available to give to the patient. (A nasal cannula should be used if oxygen is necessary). The nurse should reassure the patient and explain everything that is happening and will happen.

Hemostasis can become a problem during the procedure. The surgical nurse needs to assist in controlling bleeding by handing the appropriate instruments to the physician and applying pressure on the correct area. The nurse should also have ready the appropriate suture ligation material or electrical surgical equipment for the physician to use for hemostasis. Afterward an appropriate pressure dressing should be applied on the area, along with instructions given to the patient about what to do in case of bleeding. The patient should be told to decrease his or her activity and whether or not he or she should apply ice to the area and for how long to apply pressure in case of bleeding. The patient should also be given emergency telephone numbers to call if he or she should have any problems at home following their procedure.

The nurse must be ready for any emergency that may arise during a procedure. This includes a knowledge of basic life support and information regarding availability of emergency equipment and how to use it. Standard equipment includes an ambu bag, airway and intubation equipment, oxygen, and emergency medications. In some institutions there are code teams available to respond to emergency situations. The physician and nursing team should have an established plan of action for emergencies.

POSTOPERATIVE ASSESSMENT

Immediately after the procedure and before the patient leaves the office the nurse needs to explain wound-care instructions to the patient. The patient should receive these instructions both verbally and also in writing.[5] It is helpful if the patient is accompanied by someone who can also receive the instructions at the same time. If the doctor has prescribed an antibiotic or any type of pain medication, then it is up to the nurse to ensure that the patient understands how to take the medication. It is also important that the patient be told that he or she may experience various symptoms after their procedure, such as swelling, bruising, and discomfort; there may be a black eye (if surgery was near or above the eye). The patient should also be told how to handle these problems. The patient may use ice over the area for the first 24 to 48 hours. After that, if there is still discomfort, the patient can use heat over the area. He or she also needs to be told what to look for, such as any signs of infection. Streaking, unusual redness, pus, an unusual amount of drainage, and severe pain should all be reported to the physician.

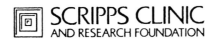

SCRIPPS CLINIC
AND RESEARCH FOUNDATION

Hubert T. Greenway, Jr., M.D.
Division of Dermatology and Cutaneous Surgery
Mohs' Chemosurgery

INSTRUCTIONS FOR POST-OPERATIVE WOUND CARE

1. Cleanse wound with hydrogen peroxide using Q-tips.
2. Dry wound with gauze and apply Bacitracin Ointment using Q-tips.
3. Cover with Telfa and gauze cut to size and apply non-allergic tape (papertape).
4. Change dressing _____ times daily.
5. You may get your wound wet after the first 24 hours. If you wish to shampoo your hair, we recommend a mild shampoo (such as Johnson's Baby Shampoo).
6. If bleeding should occur, apply 20 minutes of CONSTANT pressure.
7. Return visit: _____
8. For uncontrolled bleeding or bonafide emergencies:
   Office: (619) 554-8646
   Home:

Figure 10.4. Sample of postoperative wound care patient handout with place for home emergency phone numbers at bottom (whited out for publication)

The patient should be given emergency phone numbers so that he or she can reach the physician or nurse if need be any time of the day or night (Figure 10-4). The patient should also be given a follow-up appointment and told at that time if it will be with the nurse for a dressing change or with the physician.

If the patient comes back to see the nurse, then the nurse will assess the wound, ensuring that there are no signs of infection and reviewing the wound-care instructions again with the patient. If the patient is coming in for suture or staple removal it is help-ful if the nurse explains to the patient what will be taking place during that visit. If the patient is to use steri-strips, then it is up to the nurse to explain how to change them or whether they just need to be left in place.

CONCLUSION

When a patient comes in to see the physician for the first time, he or she may be appre-hensive and scared and may hear only half of what is being told to them during that visit. Sometimes patients do not ask any questions because they are afraid. It is up to the nursing staff to ensure that the patient understands what will take place, to explain again the procedure, and even to have the physician spend more time with the patient before the procedure.

The patient may have many fears including the possibility of disfigurement and physical appearance after surgery. The nurse must provide the patient with reassurance to help him or her through this very trying time. Our written materials may help with patient education and understanding, but it is the human touch and caring of the nurse that can provide for a successful result and a happy patient.

REFERENCES

1. Stegman SJ, Tromovitch TA. *Cosmetic Dermatologic Surgery.* Chicago, IL: Year Book Medical Publishers; 1984:2–5.
2. Roenigk RK, Roenigk HH. *Dermatology Surgery, Principles and Practice.* New York, NY: Marcel Dekker Inc.; 1989:51–61.
3. Bennett RG. *Fundamentals of Cutaneous Surgery.* St Louis, MO: CV Mosby; 1988:195.
4. Salasche SJ. Acute surgical complications: Cause, prevention and treatment. *J Am Acad Dermatol.* 15:1163–1185, 1986.
5. Scarborough DA, Bisaccia E, Swanson RD. Anesthesia for outpatient dermatologic cosmetic surgery: Midazolam—low dose ketamine anesthesia. *J Dermatol Surg Oncol.* 15:658–665, 1989.
6. Grekin R, Auletta MJ. Local anesthesia in dermatologic surgery. *J Am Acad Dermatol.* 19:599–614, 1988.
7. Winton GB. Anesthesia for dermatologic surgery. *J Dermatol Surg Oncol.* 14:41–45, 1988.
8. Auletta MJ, Grekin R. *Local Anesthesia for Dermatologic Surgery.* New York, NY: Churchill Livingstone; 1991:9–24.
9. Brown CD. Drug interactions in dermatologic surgery. *J Dermatol Surg Oncol.* 18:512–516, 1992.

PERSONAL PERSPECTIVES

Terry L. Barrett, MD*

Hubert T. Greenway, Jr. MD

INTRODUCTION

As we conclude this work on preoperative and postoperative care in dermatologic surgery we want to share with you our personal thoughts and perspectives on some common situations the physician will invariably face in clinical practice. These thoughts are not to be construed as dogma but are based on reflections of our own experience and represent our approach to dealing with these problems. It is our hope that our perspectives will serve to crystallize your thinking in similar situations that you may face in your practice.

HOW TO TALK TO PATIENTS

The patient will have a number of concerns and will make an appointment that may lead to an actual dermatologic surgical procedure. The patient may or may not have beforehand knowledge of the physician, but to provide effective care, it is important for

---

*The opinions or assertions contained herein are the private views of the authors and not to be construed as official or as reflecting the views of the U.S. Navy or the Department of Defense.

us as physicians to be interested not only in the individual's disease process but also the patient as a person. Certainly we as physicians want to make a good impression on the patient. Often, however, this can best be done by telling the patient that you are impressed by him or her.

In attempting to make the patient at ease, it is important not to underestimate small courtesies such as trying to be on time for the patient's appointment. The attitude and manner of your individual staff members will also have made an impression on the patient before your first consultation.

In dealing with the new patient, the physician develops the theme for the consultation at the beginning. Some physicians are more formal, and therefore the consultation remains in a formal state. We have found that beginning on a note of friendliness presents a more caring attitude and allows the patient to be more comfortable and at ease. Perhaps best is to allow the patient to do the verbal communication. Certainly this takes time, and time is an important commodity in the physician's everyday practice. However, patients have many apprehensions, and it is important that they be allowed to express these as they tell us their story and reason for being in our office. The spouse or any family members should be recognized and allowed to provide their input.

Because most of our patients and their family member(s)/spouse are normally in a sitting position when we enter the room, we try to conduct at least a portion of the consultation or initial interview in a sitting position, if possible. When the physician constantly looks down from a standing position, patients tend to feel smaller than they really are; in addition, sitting down gives the impression that one has adequate time for patients to fully express their feelings and concerns during that visit. A smile is an excellent way to warm up a new patient; however, a smile must be real and not phony. There is of course such a thing as being too charming. Perhaps the surest way to convince the patient that you are one of the wisest, most intelligent physicians that he or she has ever met is to listen and pay attention to what the patient has to say. The fact that you attach enough importance to what the patient is saying proves to him or her that you are a very smart and caring physician.

HOW TO DEAL WITH THE REFERRING PHYSICIAN

Many patients are referred by another physician and are grateful to that physician for assisting them in seeking specialized care. A dermatologic surgeon, in addition to providing the best possible referral care, must be able to communicate well with the physician who provided the referral. In most cases, a copy of the written consultation or operative report can be provided to the referring physician for his or her information and files. Some referring physicians have special requests such as a postoperative polaroid photograph. Others appreciate a phone call to them directly, and certain physicians in busy practices may wish to give this information to one of the staff; the information will be then relayed to the referring physician between patient visits.

It is important to commend the referring physician for care that he or she has provided and to give credit for previous treatment, establishing of the diagnosis, or care up until that point. Physicians should be generous with kind statements.

A critical step in the patient–physician relationship is for you always to return the patient to the referring physician. In most cases this is easy to do, but on occasion it may be difficult and can be a source of conflict. Our referring physicians are excellent individuals and practitioners, and we always point out to their patients that they certainly are lucky to be under his or her care. Normally, when we tell the patient the only problem we have ever heard regarding their referring physician relates to the difficulty of getting an appointment because the physician is so excellent elicits a smile; the patient is assured that we feel comfortable returning him or her to the referring physician.

HOW TO COMMUNICATE WITH THE PATHOLOGIST

Pathology is a complex specialty requiring integration of clinical situations with disease processes as they appear histologically. Ideally, a biopsy is submitted to the pathologist and a definitive diagnosis results. Often this is possible. However, many variables come into play in the histologic manifestations of disease. Sampling of a lesion by biopsy may not be representative of the disease process. Furthermore, diseases are dynamic processes and a biopsy taken only once, which may or may not be diagnostic of the overall process. Treatment may alter textbook descriptions of diseases. Often, there are many histologic patterns for a single disease depending on the site and time of the biopsy in the disease course. Conversely, many disease processes may have similar histologic findings.

It is imperative to remember that the pathologist is a physician that you are consulting for his or her expertise in this area of medicine. All relevant information should be provided at the time the tissue examination is requested. No physician should be asked to make a diagnosis without adequate information. No physician would think of doing only a physical examination without taking a history, yet it is surprising how often a pathologist is asked to do just that under the guise of being "objective." Although pathologists often enjoy looking at slides without clinical information to determine how much information they can extract from the slide (and this is a useful method to teach residents and fellows observation skills), no diagnosis should ever be made in a real situation involving the diagnosis and treatment of a patient without all information being taken into account.

The clinician can best assist the pathologist at this early stage of the consultation by ensuring that the tissue examination request form is as complete as possible, including the following information: age, sex, location of process, number of lesions, and whether multiple lesions are similar or different. Present or previous treatment should be recorded as well as the results of any previous biopsies. Most important is the clinician's judgment as to the likely differential diagnosis. Pathologists are well trained in residency programs today; however, the general pathologist must divide his or her time in training and in practice among all organ systems. The pathologist's training in dermatology is not likely to be as extensive as the clinician's submitting the specimen. Furthermore, as stated previously, the pathologist is viewing the biopsy at a fixed point in time. He or she is watching a single frame of a slide show whereas the clinician is watching the movie. The clinician's judgment of the differential diagnosis is paramount for the pathologist to provide the best possible histologic diagnosis.

Clinicians should ask themselves "What do I need to know to treat the patient? If the consideration is compound nevus versus malignant melanoma, a clinical diagnosis of rule out (r/o) melanoma may be all that is necessary. However, if the clinical consideration is recurrent nevus versus melanoma, it is absolutely critical that the history of previous treatment be communicated to the pathologist. Distinction between the various types of eczematous processes may be impossible histologically; in this case, the only pathology diagnosis possible is spongiotic dermatitis. Obviously, clinical information again is paramount.

A clinically nonspecific process will often likewise be histologically nonspecific. The pathologist may only be able to give a descriptive diagnosis until the disease manifests itself. One must remember that the pathology lab is not the Supreme Court with the pathologist as Chief Justice. Diagnoses often must be modified as diseases evolve and more information becomes available. The goal must always be to provide the best possible care to the patient and work together as a team over time. Despite your best efforts to provide a completed tissue examination form and do an adequate biopsy, there will be times when this is not sufficient and a telephone call to the pathologist is required. A telephone call is always the best course of action to alert the pathologist to an unusual case or a particular problem in advance of the surgery. The pathologist may have suggestions as to the type of biopsy, method of submission (eg, fresh tissue to lab or special fixative) that may save the patient from having to undergo an additional procedure at a later time.

Even after the clinician has received a report, telephone calls are often desirable. For example, if the pathologic diagnosis is lichen planus but the biopsy was of a single lesion on the chest to rule out basal cell carcinoma, a discussion with the pathologist regarding the entity of benign lichenoid keratosis can be quite instructive.

Communication, both written and verbal, between the clinician and the pathologist is never wasted and ultimately results in better care for the patient.

HOW TO RETRIEVE OLD SLIDES/REPORTS IN A NONTHREATENING WAY

Perhaps a pigmented lesion was previously removed by shave biopsy and has now recurred. The original diagnosis was compound nevus. Is this present lesion a recurrent nevus or is it a melanoma? Was the original diagnosis correct? Another hypothetical example: A patient was previously treated for basal cell carcinoma with electrodesiccation and curettage. The patient now presents with paresthesia along the course of a nerve present at the site. Was perineural invasion missed on the original biopsy? These situations along with many others require review of the original biopsy slides.

Pathologists are human, and like all humans, they will occasionally make mistakes. Like any physician, they are concerned with the possibility of making a mistake that results in a poor outcome. Unfortunately, pathologists' mistakes do not heal but are preserved forever on glass slides and are available for review by others. Pathologists are naturally concerned about being second-guessed. Nonetheless, there are innumerable instances that require review of old slides and reports. How does one go about requesting this information in a nonthreatening way?

Many facilities have developed their own standard form that is routinely used to request slides, blocks, or reports from laboratories. However, it may be useful to attach a cover letter explaining the nature of the request and an offer to send a copy of the pathology report from your institution following the review.

The situation can be more complicated and potentially uncomfortable when the slides were originally interpreted by the dermatologist who also provided the treatment. If this physician is the referring physician, then usually rapport has been previously established. However, if the patient is seeking a second opinion, or if the patient is presenting with a complication that may require additional treatment, there will likely be great concern on the part of the original physician. It is even more important in this case to reassure the original physician, usually with a cover letter and often a telephone call, discussing the nature of the consultation and your need for review of the original material in order to provide therapy. Again, an offer to send a copy of the pathology report from your institution and a letter summarizing your care is appreciated.

The overriding concern is to provide the best care available to the patient. All physicians, whether clinicians or pathologists, benefit from such an approach.

HOW TO SUBMIT A SPECIMEN IF SPECIAL STAINS ARE REQUIRED

Routine formalin fixation and paraffin embedding are sufficient for diagnosis of most dermatologic conditions. Most "special stains" such as periodic acid-Schiff (PAS) or silver stains and most immunoperoxidase stains can be performed on formalin-fixed, paraffin-embedded tissue. Occasionally, however, additional studies may be needed that require special handing of the tissue.

Most commonly, these fall into two special categories: specimens that require immunofluorescence (eg, lupus erythematosus, pemphigus vulgaris), and specimens in which the diagnosis of a lymphoid process is being considered (eg, lymphoma versus pseudolymphoma).

Each laboratory has its own handling requirements for these special studies, and it is best to call the pathologist before obtaining the specimen. Lymphoid processes normally require special fixation, such as B-5 fixative, which must be prepared fresh before use. Additionally, certain immunoperoxidase markers and immunofluorescence studies require frozen tissue.

Optimal utilization of tissue results from advanced planning and consultation with the pathologist.

HOW TO DEAL WITH "ATYPICAL" LESIONS: WHAT TO TELL THE PATIENT

Patients understand the word *benign* to mean a noncancerous condition that in most cases is nonthreatening. They also understand the word *malignant* to mean a condition, neoplasm, or tumor that needs to be completely and effectively treated to ensure the patients' state of health and longevity. The term *atypical* may be unsettling to them and may raise concerns regarding your methods of treatment. When such a situation arises in my (HTG) practice, I like to spend time communicating with the patient. I try to relate back to my days of practicing general dermatology when it was important for me to sit down, take out a pad, and start drawing and writing out various things for my patients with a diagnosis of atopic dermatitis. This would often include the various triggering factors, itch, scratch cycle, and certain treatment parameters as well as complications. In the case of the "atypical lesion" I also sit down and spend time with the patient, drawing out a spectrum with "benign" at one end and "malignant" at the other, with "atypical" in the center, and point out to the patient that we were fortunate enough to make the diagnosis with the lesion in an intermediary state.

Certainly we could not state that all these lesions would then progress nor can we predict an absolute time frame of progression, but in any event the diagnosis was made in an early state to the patient's benefit. In addition, second opinions regarding the pathologic diagnosis may be obtained, but most patients feel comfortable knowing that the situation was handled at an early state. In certain cases no further treatment is indicated; to ensure complete removal of an "atypical" lesion, however, further surgical care may be offered in selected cases. Just as each lesion is different, each situation is different, and it is in the patient's best interest for the physician to provide as much information as that individual patient needs, such as in the case of a patient with multiple atypical lesions.

HOW TO RESOLVE CONFLICTS IN THE INTERPRETATION OF A BIOPSY IN THE BEST INTEREST OF THE PATIENT

It has been stated that if you show a slide to 10 pathologists, you will get 10 opinions as to the diagnosis. Although it is an obvious exaggeration, this statement does underscore the subjectivity that is inherent in the specialty of pathology.

Pathologists are trained to be objective. They strive constantly to diagnose lesions using objective, reproducible criteria. As a result of their inherent subjectivity, however, pathologists will disagree on occasion regarding the diagnosis of a particular case. This can result potentially in one slide having two different diagnoses.

How should one approach this situation? Ideally, we believe that the pathologist should choose consultants in which he or she has confidence in various subspecialties. When a diagnostic problem arises, the pathologist should then seek the opinion of only one expert, and whenever possible, that opinion should be honored. Sending cases to more than one expert invariably leads to more than one diagnosis for a particular case. This forces generalists to choose which expert opinion they prefer in order to prepare their own reports. Other pathologists choose to send all diagnoses to the clinician, forcing the clinician to choose which diagnosis he or she will treat. Both situations are fraught with difficulty. A single, well-chosen expert eliminates this problem.

Nonetheless, well-founded differences of opinion will occur. In the case of inflammatory lesions, time will usually resolve the discrepancy as the disease declares itself, leading to a final well-established diagnosis. However, in the case of tumors, waiting—and thereby delaying treatment—is rarely the proper course of action.

In general, we believe that the best approach to disputes involving tumors is to ensure that the entire lesion is excised. This not only provides additional tissue for examination but gives both the clinician and the patient a sense of satisfaction that a legitimate attempt has been made to cure the lesion.

HOW TO DEAL WITH A LOST SPECIMEN

The absolute best way to deal with a lost specimen is to prevent the specimen from being lost in the first place.

Specimens may be lost before they arrive in the laboratory. One way to reduce significantly the number of lost specimens is to have the surgeon place the specimen directly in the specimen cup. At this point, the surgeon should double-check the labeling of the container. Is this the correct patient? The correct location? The surgeon can also ensure that the specimen is adequately covered with formalin. Specimens, particularly small ones, may get stuck to the side or to the lid of the container and go undetected at the time of grossing. Although this is a difficult habit to develop, particularly when you may be trying to control bleeding, it is well worth the time required. Try to keep in mind the purpose of the biopsy.

Despite all the surgeon's best efforts, specimens are occasionally lost in laboratory processing. Again, the best way to deal with this problem is to prevent it from occurring. Grossing stations that remove the grossing platform from the vicinity of running water are preferred. This type of station is ideal for small specimens such as the majority of skin specimens, as the chance that the specimen will be dropped and washed away is reduced. Wire screens are available that can cover the sink drain, resulting in a trap to catch specimens in the event that a specimen is dropped into running water.

Modern automated tissue processors also have screens that will catch small specimens in the event that the tissue cassette comes open during processing. At the time of tissue embedding, if there is no specimen in the tissue cassette, the technician simply checks this "tissue trap", recovering the specimen.

Implementing the preceding procedures will substantially reduce the incidence of lost specimens. However, despite everyone's best efforts, occasionally a specimen will be lost, improperly processed, or somehow damaged in such a way as to render a diagnosis impossible.

We believe the best approach at this point is for the pathology report to indicate that the specimen was lost (or damaged) and the pathologist should call the clinician. Physician-to-physician contact is best at these times.

The clinician should conduct another biopsy of the lesion if possible, but if no lesion remains and a malignant diagnosis was being considered, reexcision of the scar or previous biopsy site should be considered.

Just as in the previous discussion on resolving conflicts, ensuring complete removal of the lesion site, even in the absence of a histopathologic diagnosis, is in the best interest of the patient.

HOW TO PREVENT LAWSUITS

Most of us can recall our elderly professor telling us how he had never been sued in 40 to 50 years of medical practice. This is a wonderful tribute. It is doubtful that the vast majority of us will be able to survive the lifespan of a normal practice without the possibility of several legal actions. Prevention is certainly the most effective management and overall the most rewarding. In many cases what is perceived as a lack of communication and caring may be the reason that events lead to legal action. Selective hearing is the norm for the patient–physician encounter, and what the patients thinks we said may indeed be as important to him or her as what we actually did say. The ability of the physician to listen to the patient so as to care for his or her needs demonstrates that you are interested in the patient as an individual and not only an acute medical problem. In the past the failure to diagnose a melanoma had been at the forefront of medical/legal actions of dermatologists and dermatologic surgeons. However, in today's environment the patient's perception of an incompletely successful surgical outcome and problems with appropriateness of informed consent are perhaps more indicative of the typical action against our specialty.

Just as caring and communication are important in our dealings with the patient, documentation is the key to providing an adequate medical record and protecting the physician. Photographs, drawings, and a detailed medical record provide a pathway of the patient's care and demonstrate the physician's thoroughness and appropriateness of care. Even the documentation of the follow-up phone calls, although seemingly a small detail is a good idea.

On rare occasions, patients or family members may inappropriately seek your support against another physician. Indeed, in our practice at the Scripps Clinic we have even had a patient's family member go as far as to conceal a tape recorder in her purse in hopes of capturing comments that might support the patient's case. In any event, it is important always to honor our professional colleagues, and certainly if we were not present at the time of any previous medical or surgical care it would be difficult to know what that physician was thinking. It is important for us to assist and help a physician colleague whenever possible. In addition, one may wish to communicate with other physicians and keep them informed. Certainly one would not want to make an enemy of another physician and create problems. Remember that two experts can disagree, even when they are both working for the good of the patient.

Finally, in most practices it is not necessary that you be the treating physician for every patient you encounter or who is referred to you. If for some reason the doctor–patient relationship does not seem to be a good one or you have any hesitancy, it may be in both your and the patient's best interests for the two of you together to seek another physician to provide care for that patient. On occasion I hear a young dermatologic surgeon admit, "If only I had referred this patient to someone else then the medical/legal problem that arose would have been their problem and not mine." Unfortunately, such an awareness for most of us only comes after years of experience.

IN SPITE OF BEST EFFORTS—WHAT TO DO WHEN YOU GET SUED

California is often the bellwether for the rest of the United States, and this is certainly true in the medical/legal arena. In spite of our efforts, physicians continue to receive periodic notification of an impending legal action. In the past this had averaged once every six to seven years for dermatologists and dermatologic surgeons, but at the present the occurrence appears to be more frequent. Certainly we believe that the care and concerns we provide to our patients continue to be excellent and appropriate; it may be that the attitudes of society and the possibility that there is an overabundance of lawyers are contributing to the increase of medical/legal activities. Very often disbelief is the initial feeling one has the first time one is the defendant in a medical malpractice litigation case. We spend our whole lives preparing ourselves and providing appropriate care and treatment for patients; it is hard for us to believe that someone would actually seek action against us. There may be the rare case where a mistake was made or an accident occurred, but this is the exception not the norm. In certain cases (eg, alleged problems with interpretation of radiology claims, allegedly missed pathology diagnosis, or denial by managed care utilization committees), you may be named as a defendant when in reality you are only on the periphery.

Often the first step in defending against a suit is to obtain the medical chart and see exactly what has happened in the actual treatment. At this point the physician may notice minor inconsistencies or incompleteness and may be tempted to provide more information. It is most important that the chart not be altered or edited in any fashion. Even innocent attempts to provide additional information will be used against the physician. No additions or alterations to the chart whatsoever can be made. It is important, however, that the chart be placed in a secure place for safekeeping.

Once a complaint has been received, the physician should forward it immediately to his or her medical malpractice insurance carrier and lawyer. Otherwise the case should not be discussed, as any communications could then be brought forth later.

Currently it is the custom at Scripps Clinic to disengage in the medical care of that individual patient at the time that a medical/legal action is filed. The case is handled by our medical/legal staff, and in our opinion this is in the best interests of our medical staff and the patients alike.

In the event of a full process of the medical/legal action (ie, depositions, trial, and so on) the physician may experience significant stress at certain times. Certain physical activities (eg, perhaps working in a backyard garden) may be good therapy and may function to alleviate stress during this time.

Robert Cosgrove in Chapter 2 provides an excellent essay on this subject that should be read on more than one occasion by each of us. He is very supportive of his physicians during a medical defense action, and we have been fortunate to have him participate in our continuing medical education courses for physicians.

HOW TO EMPLOY ALL AVAILABLE RESOURCES

At the time of surgery we would like for our patients to be in the best of health and utilize all available resources. Appropriate physical exercise or activity (or limitations) and a good diet may be addressed preoperatively.

Dietary supplements including vitamins, antioxidants and minerals may be beneficial in both wound healing and long term maintenance. The elimination and avoidance of tobacco products and other substances which adversely affect wound healing should be encouraged.

SUMMARY

Preoperative evaluations and postoperative care can be just as rewarding as surgical procedures. The preoperative evaluation always allows a good doctor–patient relationship to be established or renewed. Postoperative visits are a time for reassurance. If there are problems, listen to the patient, participate in his or her discomfort and distress. Dealing and communicating effectively with the referring physician, the patient's other physicians (on occasion), and the pathologist allows you to perform in the patient's best interest. Becoming the patient's ally promotes a good outcome and increases the knowledge and experiences of the dermatologic surgeon.

INDEX